ANATOMY

OF

ANOREXIA

The Best Little Girl in the World

Treating and Overcoming Anorexia

Kessa

Obsessive-Compulsive Disorders

The Luckiest Girl in the World

Cutting

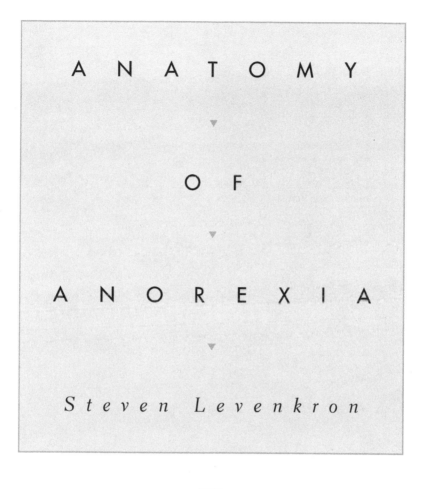

ANATOMY

OF

ANOREXIA

Steven Levenkron

W. W. NORTON & COMPANY

NEW YORK / LONDON

For information about permission to reproduce selections from this book, write to
Permissions, W. W. Norton & Company, Inc., 500 Fifth Avenue, New York, NY 10110

The text of this book is composed in Electra
with the display set in Futura
Composition by Platinum Manuscript Services
Manufacturing by Courier Westford
Book design by JAM Design

Library of Congress Cataloging-in-Publication Data

Levenkron, Stephen, 1941–
        Anatomy of anorexia / Steven Levenkron.
        p.   cm.
        Includes bibliographical references and index.
        ISBN 0-393-04835-7
        1. Anorexia nervosa Popular works. I. Title.
    RC552.A5L478   2000
    616.85'262—dc21   99-39958
                                                       CIP

W. W. Norton & Company, Inc., 500 Fifth Avenue, New York, NY 10110
www.wwnorton.com

W. W. Norton & Company, Ltd., 10 Coptic Street, London WC1A 1PU

1 2 3 4 5 6 7 8 9 0

To all those brave souls who have given up
the only security they knew, for a healthier,
frightening, unfamiliar adventure—
the quest for a richer life.

ACKNOWLEDGMENTS

WOULD like to thank the many people who helped me work through this complex subject.

These include my daughter Gabrielle who from the first page kindly but relentlessly prodded me to communicate most directly with my readers, as any good editor should. Olga Wieser, my friend, my agent of twenty-four years, and, for this book, my editor throughout, seamlessly knitted any random thoughts together and monitored me for inconsistencies inherent in the creative process. Jill Bialosky, who continues to be my editor at W. W. Norton, reads my unexpressed intentions, draws them out, and weaves them together with the readers' "need to know."

I would also like to thank my daughter Rachel who taught me how to use this computer instead of the pile of typewriters I had formerly relied on and Dr. Michael Strober, for his pshycopharmacological guidance. Finally, I would like to thank my wife of thirty-six years—and more to come—Abby, for her constant encouragement in all my work.

CONTENTS

INTRODUCTION

NOREXIA nervosa, along with all eating disorders in which victims experience drastic changes in weight and appearance, has fascinated and intrigued the public for the last twenty years. The number of new victims does not seem to be declining, and neither does the public's appetite for information as they observe the eight million victims and hear their stories.

During the last fifteen years, TV talk shows featuring anorexia have ballooned into circus sideshows, while magazine articles explore new angles on the disease and hunt down celebrities who may have it. Anorexia remains damagingly epidemic to its victims and a spectator sport for the nonafflicted public.

Perhaps the public's sometimes macabre interest is a combination of dread that daughters, sisters, wives, or friends might contract the disorder; some might be interested in the disease because their own inability to lose weight and unconscious desire to be thinner is relieved by witnessing the disaster and folly of its fulfillment; others might worry that their own obsession with thinness and weight could develop into anorexia.

Even with all the attention and interest anorexia receives, there are still unanswered mysteries: Why do people contract it? Why do so few recover? (Estimates on the number of women who recover from anorexia range from an optimistic 48 percent to a pessimistic 20 percent and lower.) Is anorexia a form of insanity? What could be so powerful about the disorder that it causes anorexics to ruin or end their lives for the sake of emaciation?

Alas, the only phrase we hear repeated over and over again is "control." We hear it on TV shows and read it in print articles all the time. But "control" is such a shallow formula that it leaves the complexity and mysteriousness of the disorder untouched. The term "control" has been misrepresented to suggest that the anorexic is seeking control over her life or over other members of her family. This misrepresentation makes her seem selfish and manipulative. In fact, "control" as used here refers to regulating one's own anxieties and maintaining a sense of mental organization.

Anatomy of Anorexia offers the reader an understanding of the origins and internal mental/emotional mind-set of the disease process. It shows an internal picture of the mental changes the disease's victims go through in their descent toward something like insanity. This disease changes its victims with every passing day. It makes them sicker. It is rarely "outgrown." I have identified stages of the illness, which are explicitly described. The reader will see the effects of heredity, chemistry, family, and social trends, and how they interact to create a nearly intractable disease.

In the last twenty years I have treated nearly three hundred anorexics and I have written about several girls in my practice. I am pleased to state that I have had a 90 percent recovery rate, though tragically, with one fatality. (The American Psychiatric Association estimates the death rate at 5–9 percent.) I define "recovery" as eliminating the obsessive preoccupation to weigh less than medically accepted levels, and setting realistic goals about eating and appearance, which then results in a gradual resumption of normal weight and eating patterns.

The new health care requirements have severely reduced the options of extended hospitalizations and outpatient psychotherapy benefits. This change puts more of the burden on the family's participation in the anorexic's recovery. The positive change since 1989 is the introduction of Prozac, followed by Zoloft, Paxil, Effexor, Luvox, Celexa, Serzone, and more new medications to assist patients in their recovery, coupled with effective psychotherapy.

Twenty years ago, anorexia was known to a few clinicians and researchers in psychiatry and psychology. Today, everyone from the supermarket checker to the fellow pumping gas seems to have heard of it.

We have written accounts dating back to the twelfth century of individuals displaying symptoms of what is clearly anorexic behavior. Vatican files list over one hundred cases of women who have been canonized for what seemed to be extremely virtuous behavior, working themselves to death while giving their food to others (Bell, 1989). Yet anorexia has never been seen as a commonplace illness. In the past, the disease was considered too rare to measure the commonalities between anorexic cases. It is only since the 1970s that we have seen anorexia reach its current epidemic numbers—one in every two hundred and fifty girls, according to the American Psychiatric Association (DSM IV).

Why has anorexia become an epidemic among girls? Why as a society are we so fascinated by it? Anorexia nervosa is about the influence of the fashion industry's role in shaping women's bodies, about women hating their bodies, and about family dysfunctional dynamics, resulting from societal pressures on parents not to prolong childhood dependency for as long as is necessary for each child. Perhaps above all, anorexia nervosa is about the competition among women for physical perfection, whatever that may mean.

An inability to form attachments, and a dependency between child and parent that in turn prevents healthy attachments between the child and anyone else in her life, are undoubtedly the pervasive characteristics among anorexic victims. Anorexia is not the only manifestation of this lack of attachment. Obsessive-compulsive disorders, phobias, obsessionally rigid personalities, and perfectionism in general are other disorders that both men and women develop as a result of family dysfunctions and insufficient attachment.

With at least eight million victims of eating disorders in the United States, and double that number who could be considered "subclinically eating-disordered," we are certainly looking at a cultural phenomenon. Ninety-five percent of anorexics are women. There is a clear message that women should be thin. This message is beamed to every girl and woman who reads magazines, goes to the movies, or watches television.

To understand the staying power of anorexia, one only has to look at the pictures in women's service and fashion magazines from the past twenty years, imagining the impact of the fashion industry on impressionable girls. Or at female stars in feature films and TV dramas, and topics on talk shows. Or at the diet and physical fitness industry. Girls growing up in our society are made aware as early as the age of five that adequacy, and thus acceptance, means "thin." Today's girls are the second generation growing up with this message. They are the first, however, to receive it not only from the media but also from observing their mothers and older sisters worrying about gaining weight.

It is naturally inherent in femininity to try to be alluring to men in order for the species to mate and reproduce. The standard of femininity is determined by societal norms of feminine allure. In centuries past, for example, more corpulent women were considered the most attractive. Women aspired to that appearance. In our society today, the woman with the least amount of fat tissue is considered the most alluring. This is society's message to women, not to men. For men to be considered attractive to women, they should be tall (not easily alterable after early adolescence), have a full head of hair, and earn a good income. Much of masculine allure is not cosmetic, despite media emphasis on being "ripped, cut, and buffed." Men rarely believe that their physical appearance is important in attracting women, any more than they believe that they have to look young. Men may become workaholics, seek power over others at work, or buy expensive status cars to attract women. Consequently, men constitute only 5 percent of anorexia sufferers. The men I have treated for anorexia have, for a variety of reasons, identified with society's message to women, been severely obsessive-perfectionistic, and/or suffered from other severe psychiatric disorders as well. Otherwise, male anorexia runs the same course as female anorexia.

There have been two major changes in the treatment of eating disorders in the past sixteen years, since the publication of my book, *Treating and Overcoming Anorexia Nervosa* (1982). The first is the introduction and use of new medications that stimulate the brain's use of serotonin. The second is the change in health care policies: specifically, the restriction of the use of hospitalization for anorexia nervosa patients, leaving hapless parents and families to deal with this dangerous, frightening, and divisive illness at home. Any new book in this field will have to assist parents in becoming actively involved in the treatment at home. They will need a theoretical model of the illness that makes sense to them, a cursory familiarity with medications available today, and an ethical guide to using them.

What follows is a road map outlining the medical, physical, cultural, familial, and psychological aspects of the disease process itself. My sources are the sufferers themselves—the girls and women I have treated over the past twenty-five years, ever since that first frighteningly thin fourteen-year-old entered my office with an esoteric diagnosis of anorexia nervosa. The major aim of this book is to help you identify the anorexic in your life before it is too late, and to show you what you can do to assist in her recovery. As a therapist who treats anorexic individuals, I've been asked by clinicians and the general public, "What causes it?" It is my hope that this book will help demystify this life-ruining disease.

ANATOMY

OF

ANOREXIA

1

EARLY BEGINNINGS

O BVIOUSLY, not all girls and women exposed to our cultural emphasis on thinness develop eating disorders. A large majority of them remain healthy. We are reassured when we can name one or two factors that will determine whether or not someone will develop anorexia. Although realistically we cannot identify the factors that tilt the balance in favor of illness or health, we do know that the years between puberty and young adulthood—ages eleven to twenty-two—are the most vulnerable for the onset of anorexia nervosa.

In his classic work *Childhood and Society* (1950), Erik Erikson describes the two major personality struggles in adolescence as "identity versus role diffusion" and "intimacy versus isolation." The classification is very useful in understanding why some adolescents fail to negotiate their adolescence without developing psychological disorders, while others succeed. Erikson also tells us that long before the child ever encounters these struggles, as an infant he or she faces only one battle: "trust versus mistrust."

So, while we can't find one catch-all as a criterion for determining susceptibility to anorexia nervosa, we can use three of Erikson's "eight stages of life":

Trust: Dependency and attachment
Identity: Emerging from successful trust and intimacy
Intimacy: Connection with others

When small children develop a sense of trust, and later a sense of intimacy or closeness to others, and a sense of self or identity, they are not vulnerable to becoming "creatures of the culture" in its most extreme form as exemplified by the media: magazines, movies, and so on. But individuals who are seduced by popular trends allow these trends to define much of their identity.

Trust is the primary building block for identity and intimacy. Basic trust is, of course, developed during infancy, when children learn that the caretakers they depend on are safe, consistent, and dependable. This translates into "I am safe because I am fed and changed, held and rocked." It may later take the form of "I am safe because I am in someone's arms, on someone's lap," or "I see those familiar feet and legs nearby." How often we've been amused by a toddler's eager grip of the wrong jean-clad leg, in a crowded store, much to the surprise of the stranger—and the toddler.

Many situations can interfere with the development of basic trust. Some of them may be familial: illness or even the death of the mother soon after childbirth; chronic illness of another family member that uses up the family's nurturance; divorce, leaving the child with a parent suffering from feelings of abandonment; loss of the original caretaker or nanny; or a primary caretaker who doesn't behave lovingly toward the child. Inherited and biological tendencies in a child involving depression and anxiety in the child's nervous system can also interfere with the consistent flow of nurturing and structuring behavior, effectively drowning out all the goodwill, love, and energy of the parent determined to raise the child securely.

If, for whatever reason, the development of childhood trust, dependency, and attachment fails, the child must reassure herself, regulate her own anxiety, and invent a false premature independence grounded in the self-assurance of a child by a child. Children who are forced to parent or nurture themselves are the children who do not trust adults because they were not shown the comfort of a consistent nurturing flow.

Just as young children prefer simple primary colors and learn to appreciate subtle earth colors only as they grow up, so does the mistrusting child prefer black or white viewpoints; there is no room for shades of gray. This often results in the mistrusting child becoming a perfectionist, succeeding without feeling pride, the "A" student who feels like a "C" student. Self-esteem seems unattainable. The child is often inconsolable about losses or defeats experienced by any member of the family. More often than not, the child displays obsessive or perfectionist behavior.

Some of these traits, such as perfectionist behavior, may disguise themselves as gifts to parents. They may see the child as independent, not needing much support in a family overburdened by other problems. A successful child who often does well in school and is socially outgoing does not appear worrisome.

As this child reaches puberty, she may interpret her developing breasts and her menstrual periods as signaling the end of an incomplete childhood. She may feel that she must turn away from her family to complete that childhood and seek some sort of an identity for herself. Most, if not all, adolescents, turn outside or rebel against some of their family values to assert their own independence. The child who has never successfully developed a healthy dependence in her early years has nowhere to go emotionally for fulfillment of her need to develop a sense of identity but to the larger culture and its messages to girls and women. Most of those messages are about being thin and ridding oneself of unnecessary and unwanted fat. She, of all her peers, becomes the ultimate devotee of this cultural message. Glance at any issue of a women's service magazine; look at the figures of popular models, and the female television and film stars, and you'll see quite slender women with prematurely lined faces, indicating that their weight is unhealthily low.

Messages stressing normal weight as attractive and healthy are drowned out by the barrage of "the Thin Message."

The girl who doesn't get anorexia nervosa as a child has developed a healthy use of dependency and trusts her parents to moderate the extreme impulses that all adolescents experience. She is not to be seduced by the bizarre messages our culture sends out to adolescents in terms of dress styles, sexual behavior, and other demands in the area of antisocial characteristics and unrealistic roles for women.

The girl who is *not* able to reach out to her parents for refuge from these often-frightening cultural demands is left to her own devices when choosing her particular route to identity and security. *A child who becomes anorexic is using her body to express her need for perfectionism.*

However, not all anorexia nervosa cases occur at puberty. Puberty is only the first of many "separating points" that may cause some sort of crisis in girls. Other identifiable crisis junctures can happen during the junior year of high school (when exploring the option of leaving home for college), during the senior year of high school (when preparing to leave home), during the freshman year of college (when girls are living out of the home), upon graduation from college (moving further from the dependence of family life), and at other profound positive or negative life-changing moments that may occur in a young woman's life—marriage, childbirth, incest, or the loss of a best friend. These "separating points" refer to separation from a previous, less mature level of dependency, which has been unfulfilling, so that the person is unable to move on toward more independence. This derails the negotiation of Erikson's key crises of:

1. Basic trust vs. mistrust
2. Identity vs. role diffusion
3. Intimacy vs. isolation (or obsessiveness)

In the chapters that follow, the development of identity and intimacy will be discussed with regard to fostering or preventing the development of anorexia nervosa. When an individual is overwhelmed by relational or circumstantial changes in her life, she will either rely on the storehouse of strength and support built up in the past and turn to others for support, or she will turn inward, away from realistic solutions and toward psychological symptoms and disorders. Tragically, anorexia nervosa has become prominent among the disorders of "choice" our culture offers.

2

IDENTITY:

WHO INVENTS US?

C HILDREN begin life as wordless anthropologists. They study their adults' world and react to it as if it were the only truth. They dare not disbelieve their caretakers—whether parents, a nanny, an aunt, older sister, or sometimes (but rarely) a father, grandfather, stepfather, or uncle. These caretakers either look children in the eye or they don't; they are glad to see them or they are not; they seem interested in children or not; they touch them softly or harshly; they speak softly or harshly or rarely. Grown-ups are content or discontented. They are cheery sometimes, always, or never.

Children believe that adults command them. They, the children, feel responsible for their parents' attitudes toward them. If children behave well, they will be loved; if they don't, they won't. In a child's eyes, grown-ups are never wrong. Children know who they are by the manner in which adults react to them. Sometimes, children help adults to get along with each other. Sometimes, children have to cheer and support adults. They do a good job and grown-ups love them for it. Sometimes, adults love children just for being who they are. Sometimes, adults love children for what they do for them. Although children encounter many different types of adults, one thing is constant: *children study adults closely to know who they themselves are.*

In the most concrete terms, parents need to help their children experience life, and this orientation begins when adults focus on the child. Frequent, loving eye contact from parent to child tells the child, on a nonverbal level, that the child is interesting and valuable to the parent. This leads to the development of self-esteem. In addition to eye contact, voice tone is the second cue to children about how they are regarded by the parent. The child looks for warmth, confidence, and authoritativeness in the tone of the parent's voice. As children grow older, they will interpret the words that accompany the eye contact and the voice tones to develop further ideas and feelings about how they are seen by their parents.

Children like to hear that they are pretty, interesting, clever, smart, and so on. Children are demonstrative; they hug and kiss adults, tell adults that they love them. These adults might be parents, older siblings, grandparents, guardians, or anyone children believe and trust. And children will be pleased, displeased, or confused by what they observe in adults. If children hear good things about themselves, they will feel good about themselves. If they hear bad things about themselves, they will feel bad about themselves. If, however, children hear good things about themselves but don't believe them, it won't help them feel better. Worse, if children don't hear anything about themselves, or even feel that their adult models are looking to them for support, they will become invisible. Invisible, because they are lacking the identity messages that are so crucial in forming a young personality, that "fill up" the child with a sense of self. A self contains character traits, habits, behaviors, in other words, a personality. Children who are not given this support are left "undescribed," and they replace their lack of identity the only way they know how: they construct a false one to fool those around them.

Identity formation is a gamble, to be sure. The "nature-nurture" debate will no doubt continue as new DNA information is interpreted and reinterpreted to determine whether character traits are genetically inherited or formed by families. Regardless, what *is* formed by families and family systems is the way that children relate to adults—what children see, observe, and hear.

Family members are continually giving "identity messages" to each other. Children usually receive these messages from their parents, but older siblings may send them messages (often negative) as well. The younger child who goes to play with his older brother and has the older brother's bedroom door slammed in his face repeatedly learns he is unwanted, and in turn he processes this by thinking or perceiving that he is unlikable. These identity messages, if they are consistently repeated, form children's first sense of who they really are: their initial identity. If the messages are directly spoken to the child, it is a simple matter for the child to believe what is said. If the message has to be inferred (or invented) by the child, it will be negative. For example, if a child is never told that she is pretty, or smart, or isn't listened to attentively, she will always believe that she is ugly, or unfeminine, unintelligent, and boring. Parents should never assume that their children will believe that they possess positive attributes that parents have not frequently ascribed to them. There is an old (untrue) parental admonition that begins with "I don't have to tell you that you're pretty, smart, interesting, or for that matter that I love you." Children have no ability to *infer* an unstated positive parental thought about their appearance and/or their personality.

I recall an attractive nineteen-year-old in my office who described how ugly she felt she was: "My hips are too wide," "My nose is crooked," "I could use an undershirt instead of a bra." All of her comments were distortions about her face and body, but she *felt* they were real. She stated these remarks with intense self-contempt. She was not looking for reassurances. When her mother came to drive her home, I invited her into my consultation office. I asked her if she thought her daughter was plain-looking or pretty. She promptly replied: "Of course she's pretty. Why, she's beautiful!" I asked her if she ever told her daughter that she thought she was beautiful. She responded: "No, I never wanted her to get a swelled head."

Children are rarely, if ever, spoiled by compliments that are sincere. They need all the support that they can get, whether it's about their appearance, intelligence, character, or personality. That does not mean that by positively reinforcing our children, we give them unrealistic, grandiose ideas about themselves. It means that we must explicitly support the positive qualities they do have.

Most corporate supervisors' handbooks advise that before a supervisor criticizes a subordinate, that supervisor first states what the subordinate does well before executing the criticism. As parents are so frequently called upon to correct their children, they may not always have time for a positive review of the child's good qualities. That is why it is important to state them when an opportunity presents itself, so that the child will have a backlog of praise to be able to hear, tolerate, and withstand the criticism, rather than using it to confirm a general sense of being no good.

For the growing child, then, those aspects of that child that are directly spoken about are believed (even when the child acts defiant and disbelieving). Those aspects of her that are not commented on are inferred by the child to be negative. No child ever thinks, "I'm smart, I'm interesting, I'm attractive. My parents just forgot to ever mention it."

Biological Depression and Anxiety

When a child is diagnosed by a trained professional as being clinically depressed or anxious, aside from contending with that child's lack of enthusiasm, unhappiness, excessive nervousness, fearfulness, and timidity, parents will need to understand that their child believes that he or she is different from other children, that his or her mind does not work the same way. For children, "different is inferior." If family dynamics are examined in psychological evaluation by professionals and seem healthy—the family members are open and honest, the parents (if married) have a substantially caring relationship, no extraordinary emotional relationship problems are apparent to account for unhappiness or long-term frustration or feelings of nature—and don't account for the depression or anxiety in a child, and especially if there is a history of family members showing symptoms of the same problems, then a diagnosis of "chemical," "biological," or "hereditary" causes is concluded. Sometimes this kind of diagnosis results in the suggestion that medication be used as part of treatment. Usually in these cases, which vary from individual to individual, especially with children, a combination of individual psychotherapy and medication is the treatment most effective in helping a child through depression. Separate psychotherapy with the child's parents addressing and coping with the depression, or joint family therapy including the child, may be recommended.

Hereditary and psychological anxiety, and depression, all affect a child's developing sense of identity. The child will discredit the good things said about her, regardless of how much trust she has in her parents. Her parents will need to compete with the depression or anxiety continuously in order to prevent additional disorders common with young women, such as eating disorders, obsessive-compulsive disorders, agoraphobia, and crippling feelings of inferiority along with extremely poor self-esteem. It's a vicious cycle: disorders have a negative impact on identity, and negative identity creates new disorders which further devalue self-esteem.

An example: Susie is an anxious child, who is hesitant to participate in sports activities at school. When other children tease her, she feels depressed and ashamed. She develops psychosomatic disorders and hypochondria in order to stay away from school. She begins to view herself as sickly and physically weaker than other children. Her family has a no-win choice in front of them: disregarding her complaints would mean they don't believe her, thus adding to an already negative identity inventory (that collection of ideas the child has about herself); believing her would only further convince Susie that her physical condition is real. She develops psychosomatic stomachaches, causing her family grave concern: the consequences could lead to food phobias and more attention to her problems by the family.

Susie now has enough attention from her family to compensate for the low esteem in which her schoolmates hold her. Any kind of attention may be preferable to low self-esteem. Her sense of identity is drawn from negative attention and feelings of inferiority, but she is accustomed to this familiar pattern of relationships. Like most people, when it comes to relationships, Susie seeks out the familiar ways in which she is treated and regarded by other members of her family, no matter how bad these may be, rather than the unfamiliar, which could be disorienting and uncomfortable.

Chemically caused disorders (disorders caused by malfunctioning amines between brain cells—serotonin, to name but one) can cause children to have bad feelings about themselves and to invent explanations for them. They may think of themselves as inferior, or mean, or stupid. They may then act out these character and personality traits to get the family to reflect on them, or to verify them. This won't be deliberate on the child's part, but will be an attempt to make sense out of his or her feelings. Not only is it a vicious cycle when chemical disorders spur on psychological disorders in the individual, but the cycle can infect the entire family system and set of relationships.

To return to our original example, if Susie now has developed what seems to be a digestive disorder initially caused by anxiety, which has led her to become hypochondriacal and develop stomach problems, her parents are "used to it" and behave with a combination of sympathy, suspicion, and resentment. Susie becomes accustomed to being treated this way. It is certainly an improvement from the way she is treated in school, and she learns how to manipulate the sympathy, negate the suspicion and resentment, in what becomes a daily pattern of which no one is consciously aware.

Making the family "aware" of the situation is a more difficult process than simply pointing it out to them; one cannot make them understand their unconscious feelings and actions merely by telling them what these are. Susie and her family must be helped to believe in the interpretation for it to effect a change in how she feels about herself, which in turn can effect a change in her behavior.

When Susie's parents become angry, Susie feels badly about herself. When they see the effects of their anger upon her, they replace anger with guilt and kinder behavior. Susie reacts by feeling better about herself. But when Susie's parents realize that their forced kindness inhibits them from disciplining Susie, they feel resentful toward Susie, the source of their guilt and guilt-driven kindness. They become angry all over again. The parents are caught in a roller-coaster cycle of anger–guilt–resentment. Their daughter keeps herself protected from the hostile "dips" in their roller-coaster ride, makes them "pay" more by countering with higher inclines or guilty paybacks for their previously expressed anger or frustration. All of this moves Susie further and further away from peer friendships at school; since she is so involved with the developing system at home, she is less involved with developing appropriate friendships at school.

Susie's identity development is not invested in healthy social growth but in defensive behavior, in a passive-aggressive struggle with her parents. On a deeper level, she is ashamed of this and hates herself for it. So shame and self-hatred have become part of her identity.

This entire scenario I've described began with a chemical/biological/hereditary tendency toward excessive anxiety. Why would we not want Susie merely treated with medication that would make the anxiety go away? The two most obvious reasons are: (1) Susie would feel inferior taking pills just to be normal; and (2) before the emergence of anxiety can be identified, she has already developed negative psychological attitudes toward herself for being frightened and timid.

Nature — Heredity — vs. Nurture — Family and Childhood Experience

Using Susie's history as an example, we are left with the old question, Which came first, the chicken or the egg? "Came first" is the key phrase here. Everyone interested in human personality development sooner or later becomes involved in the "nature-nurture" controversy. Are we merely a genetic map? Or are we the product of our upbringing? Without attempting an in-depth discussion of this question, I would like to suggest that there are probably clusters of inherited personality traits that still remain to be identified. Shy and withdrawn, quick-tempered and impatient, are among the most obvious. Two of these "primary clusters" will probably turn out to be related to levels of anxiety and depression. There are already different chemical processes and neuroreceptors identified as responsible for both anxiety and depression. At least a half dozen medications, all developed in the last few years, can be helpful to a high percentage of patients who take them. Educated guessing is still the method of prescribing which medication will help whom. No test of the central nervous system has yet been developed to determine which chemical process would best be treated by which drug. Many questions still remain to be answered: Can life experiences from infancy onward affect the brain's chemical development, and to what degree? Or is the chemical map complete the day an infant is born?

In addition to these complex questions there remains the most nagging question, Which came first, the nature or the nurture? If the answer turns out to be "nature/heredity," exaggerated or minimized by nurture, then we can develop a method of understanding that will combine medication used for the "nature/hereditary" piece of the problem and appropriate psychotherapy to deal with the "nurture/family development." The third part of the problem is the effects of the disease process in complicating and worsening the illness. This is the model I will use to explain the causes, mental and emotional processes, and treatments for anorexia nervosa. They may apply to other disorders as well.

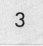

3

THE FOUR STAGES OF ANOREXIA

N order to explain anorexia, we can divide the progress of the disorder into four stages. These stages trace the disease as the victim's thoughts, feelings, and personality become distorted and her basic individuality as a person is lost, not to return until her recovery.

But first we need to clarify what anorexia is. Many descriptions of anorexia take a medical standpoint, detailing the effects that the disease's progress has on the body. Medically, anorexia is characterized by weight loss, followed by lowered body temperature, lowered blood pressure, slowed heart rate, loss of menses, thinning of hair, fatigue, and other signs of malnutrition. As the anorexic continues to lose weight, new symptoms develop and intensify. The last, lethal stage for anorexic patients is failure of the liver, kidneys, and finally, the heart.

A second way to describe the progress of anorexia is by the actions or behaviors of the victim that cause the weight loss. As the disease progresses, the anorexic consumes fewer and fewer calories. Exercise may intensify. Additional weight-losing efforts such as laxative abuse to "wash foods out" and diuretics to dehydrate the body (creating the false perception of even lower weight) are employed. All of this, combined with an unreasonable fear of protein-containing foods and attempts to replace sugar with artificial sweeteners, results in a severely malnourished, protein-deficient, overexercised, undermuscled self-starver.

Neither of these descriptions completely captures what anorexia looks like to the girl who suffers from it, nor do they answer the most important question: why is anorexic behavior so difficult to stop? The four stages of the disease that I will describe incorporate both the physical and the psychological trauma of the disease, demonstrating that these two views of anorexia cannot be separated from each other. Rather, what is *happening* to the girl's body and what the girl is *doing* to her body feed off of each other. Untreated, the chain of cause and effect could eventually kill her.

Stage One: The Achievement Stage

Anorexia typically begins with a desire on the part of the anorexic to lose weight, to be thin, and thus make herself socially acceptable to her peers. The first stage of the disease does not indicate abnormal behavior. Rather, it is in line with the trend most girls adopt who consider gaining weight unacceptable and an enemy to be fought with an all-out assault.

The majority of normal or overweight people find that dieting is depressing and boring, and deprives them of one of life's great pleasures. Most quit dieting before reaching their goals. Others who stick with their diet eventually revert to their old habits and gain back the weight they have so painfully lost. The majority of dieters are not emotionally predisposed toward anorexia. The person predisposed toward anorexia nervosa is a perfectionist, and the goal of losing weight becomes an all-consuming effort that results in "superdieting."

As the perfectionistic dieter continues to lose weight, she is at first rewarded with declarations of praise, admiration, and envy from others: "I find it so hard to lose weight; I don't know how you do it," or, "I wish I had your figure. I always quit dieting before I reach my goal."

Her sense of achievement quickly reinforces her restrictive eating pattern. Hunger pangs seem a small price to pay for the inner feelings of virtue and success, and often are interpreted as proof of success.

Stage Two: The Security-Compulsive Stage

The second stage starts with the loss of two pounds a week as a goal. The concept of "goal weight" disappears. The thinner the anorexic gets, the fatter she feels. She has crossed the border into psychopathology, or mental illness. She becomes preoccupied with measuring her arms, waist, thighs, trying on smaller sizes of clothing, and thinking about little else. She looks at every other girl her age and imagines she is fatter than they are. This "body-size distortion" is invented by her in order to maintain the mission to lose weight. If she can pretend to herself that she is fat, she can believe it is crucial to be a "fat-fighter," and this will become an important part of her impoverished sense of identity.

It is this thought that drives her on to intensify her weight-losing behaviors. She may walk more, add unreasonable amounts of stressful exercises like climbing additional flights of stairs, or use a StairMaster and other exercise machines to excess. She may increase her weight loss goal to more than two pounds a week, unlike the normal dieter, seeing each pound lost as an indicator that she needs to lose even more, as if she were gaining weight by mistake. All other girls and women seem to be thinner than her, regardless of the reality.

Her compulsion to lose weight becomes the focus. It is as if all other problems, and her relationships, have faded and her only problem is to lose weight. It becomes an *obsession*, something she is almost always thinking about. Because it has become an obsession, she must continue to find refuge in weight loss in order to reduce her anxiety. She is compelled to use her weight-losing behavior over and over again to regulate her obsessional fears, real or not, which can overwhelm her with anxiety. So she repeats the patterns compulsively to ward off her anxieties, which always feel two steps behind her.

All of this mental activity leaves little time for friends and family. The anorexic has begun to detach herself emotionally from others as she turns inward in her struggle against her body's hunger. This hunger is her brain's message that to lose more weight will result in the body's inability to use calories to keep her warm and energetic, to maintain muscle tissue, a normal heart rate, and blood pressure. Skin wrinkles develop in the crook of her arm and behind her knees, or where her arm meets her shoulder. She mistakes them for fat. In fact, these wrinkles indicate that she has shrunk her body more than her skin can contract. Her skin has become like an over-size sweater, with folds.

As she becomes thinner, the anorexic is unable to think about anything but food, day and night. The brain adapts to what it perceives as the famine conditions that must exist in her environment. Her brain wants her to become a nonstop food forager. She develops sleep disorder, haunted by thoughts of food and eating. Like her confusion about the skin folds, she mistakenly believes that she has developed an appetite that will make her obese if she gives in to it. Her brain is trying to signal her mind to save herself from death by starvation. In her confusion, she redoubles her efforts to curb her already meager intake of both food and drink. Most anorexics become liquid- as well as food-phobic.

The number of phobias mounts up: fat phobia, food phobia, weight gain phobia, appetite increase phobia, and slower metabolism phobia. This last item relates to a realistic change in the amount of calories the body burns every day. While someone is losing weight, or if they have reached a starvation weight, the body burns fewer calories per pound in its attempt to keep the person alive until the next harvest, or the next successful hunt, when food will be available again in sufficient quantities. When the body does this, it resorts to economy measures. Calories are not wasted to keep one's body temperature at 98.6 degrees Fahrenheit, so the person is cold all the time. Calories are not wasted to keep blood pressure up to normal, so dizziness often occurs. Calories are not wasted to maintain a normal heartbeat, so the heart shrinks and the number of beats per minute diminishes. Protein stores are decreasing, so the body doesn't waste protein on such nonessentials as growing scalp hair, which often becomes thinner. The menstrual cycle requires many calories and protein, and iron, so the body actually discontinues many of its vital functions in order to preserve life.

All of these body changes unfortunately are misinterpreted by the anorexic. All she understands is that now she is calorically cheaper to feed, which translates into "I have a larger appetite, I eat less despite it, and I don't lose weight. If I give in to this appetite, I will gain weight until I become obese."

How is she to find shelter and security from these fears? Eating even less and exercising have become her only solutions to achieve security. Her obsession with achieving security from these fears leads to ever-expanding protective behaviors she feels compelled to perform.

Stage two then is really an increasingly desperate attempt to *avoid insecurity,* which is doomed to failure. It will leave our victim obsessive, compulsive, distanced from others, ashamed, and depressed at her state of mind.

Stage Three: The Assertive Stage

Often, girls who develop anorexia have a history of being nice, protective, compliant, agreeable, avoiding conflict—not assertive outside their immediate family (where some of them are tyrants). The third stage develops when the girl with anorexia has been criticized for becoming too thin by many around her. She has disregarded their advice, and now their demands to stop losing weight and to start gaining are renewed.

At some point she realizes that for the first time in her life she has become defiant to everyone around her. She is no longer afraid of conflict. She is not worried about what anyone else thinks about her actions. She feels no obligation to please them. She is aware, however, that she is comfortable with this newfound defiance only in defense of her anorexia.

She does at least unconsciously feel a new sense of empowerment, even if it's only in this one limited area. It has become the most important area of her life. Outwardly, she demonstrates to her family that she has reached the third stage when she begins to demand special conditions before she will eat. For example, she may drag her parents from restaurant to restaurant, seeking the perfect, fat-free menu or dish. At home, she may stand over whoever is cooking, to make sure no extra calories are secretly added to her meal. She becomes argumentative about what she should weigh, about seeing herself as fat while others see her as too thin.

Inwardly, she believes that other women are jealous of her willpower and thinness and want her to become fat. She becomes increasingly strident in her anger when her wishes related to eating conditions are violated. She may complain "I can't eat when you're in the kitchen." This may progress to, "I can't eat when you are within sight of the kitchen, or within earshot of it." If parents follow these tyrannical dictates, they can literally end up ordered to the garage while their daughter eats.

Parents feel frightened if they disobey her, lest she lose more weight. They have no previous experience in confronting her since she has always been well behaved. Their daughter, on the other hand, is excited by her newfound assertiveness. She finds a new voice within herself, a voice that she has longed for, an assertive voice. She is aware that this voice can be used only in defense of her anorexic behavior and defying opinions about her appearance as expressed by others. When it comes to other issues, and away from home, she is still that meek, cheerful, compliant person she always was, though her sense of humor and outgoing behavior at school or work will have become overshadowed by her constant vigilance over food and weight.

This assertive stage alerts parents to the tenacity of the illness, and is the outward indication that the nightmare of anorexia has begun in earnest. Their daughter, on the other hand, is pleased, indeed, thrilled with her newfound voice. The disease has given her a new sense of power she did not anticipate when she first began to lose weight. Her *special thinness* has become one with her *special assertiveness*. To give up one would be to lose the other.

Stage Four: The Pseudo-Identity Stage

Sooner or later the anorexic's weight loss becomes obvious to the family and the community and they adapt by learning to "accept" it. Anorexia offers no privacy. Some victims hide their special thinness with layers of clothing; others are proud of it and exhibit it by exposing as much of their bodies as possible: short pants, tank tops in the summer and tight leggings in the winter. This exhibitionism becomes a weapon—an outward declaration of war against other girls and women to make a statement about who has the most willpower, who can best control her appetite. Perhaps this explains the hostility that some women feel when confronted with exhibitionistic thinness. While friends and neighbors view the "vanishing girl" with frustration and worry, others are antagonized by the pathological competitiveness. But all of them—friends, teachers, physicians, clergypersons, counselors, relatives—are referring to her as "the anorexic." Regardless of their response, whether it is anger, worry, or frustration, they all *react*. She has now achieved what she believes to be her identity, a way of being known as special, as defined. This pseudo-identity fills in the emptiness she has secretly felt about herself for some time.

This fourth stage is not characterized by new behaviors, but rather by the anorexic's new sense of power, of her own notoriety, which has marked a deepening conviction that she is on the right path. She now feels that her personality has an effect and is clearly defined by others. She prizes the newfound definition. But her "accomplishments" are rarely appreciated on a conscious level. She would no doubt object to these descriptions and generalizations, which make her sound scheming and manipulative. She may be aware of none of them.

Helping her gently and sensitively become aware of her needs and the pathological attempts she has committed herself to is the work of psychotherapy. Helping her find alternative, healthier ways to attain ends for her needs involves the development of special trust and special attachment for those who would help her.

Why does this disease deepen? Why don't its victims simply outgrow it? Although a small minority do recover without help from others, it is estimated by some authorities that as many as 70 percent never recover completely, and that the death rate from anorexia nervosa may be as high as 9 percent.

The answer may be found in the nature of the disorder. As the disease progresses, it becomes *more valuable* to the personality, despite what is lost in terms of health, relationships, and real achievements. Anorexia begins with a desire to be thin, a need to feel secure, to eliminate self-doubts and poor self-esteem, along with worries about the future. The result of anorexic behavior produces a sense of assertiveness and identity. To recover from anorexia nervosa would mean to temporarily lose one's self, to lose everything achieved by the illness.

4

OBSESSIONAL ORIGINS

IN

ANOREXIA NERVOSA

PEGGY

P EGGY was five foot five and weighed eighty-five pounds. She stood in front of the full-length mirror in my office. Her posture was not that of a person trying to see herself at her best. She slouched, thrusting her stomach out and pulling her chin into a folded-in chest. She accentuated the "S" curve of her back. She pressed her hands against the backs of her thighs.

"Look—look how fat I am! Look at my thighs! Look at my stomach!"

I was fascinated by the enormous effort she expended to create an unflattering and inaccurate representation of herself for the mirror and for me. I smiled. She was frustrated with me. "Well, can't you see the fat?"

"When I look at myself in the mirror," I said, as playfully as I could, "I stand as straight as I can, minimizing my stomach and maximizing my chest and shoulders. I pose to see myself in the best possible way. When you look at yourself in the mirror, you try to see yourself in the dumpiest possible way. I could do the same thing you did [imitating her posture], but why would I want to see myself at my worst? Why would you?"

"I'm just a realist. I don't try to disguise what's there."

"No, you're *not* a realist. You're *posing* in that mirror, creating an unflattering image to fight. You distort your spine, flatten your skinny thighs from behind to make them look dangerously wide to you, and pretend that the wrinkles on your elbows, knees, and underarms are fat. Your skin is like an oversized sweater. You've shrunk so much that it can't shrink anymore, so it wrinkles up at your limb joints. You don't dare see yourself as too thin, or even thin enough, because then you would have no reason for being. You would lose your identity as a 'fat-fighter.' And then you won't know what to do with yourself, what to think about, what to fear, what to wish for. I'm sure you would find it terrifying to view yourself as you really are. If we took away your fear of being on the edge of too fat, what would you have to think about?"

She shrugged her shoulders, retreating for the moment. "But I *am* too fat," she attempted meekly. She began to repeat this as if it were a chant. With each repetition, her voice became a little stronger. She was turning away from my reality and inward to support her own obsessional reality.

Why did she turn inward? It seems to us like a foolish choice and certainly not in her best interest. In the absence of interpersonal attachments, Peggy had become *self-stimulating*. She had invented her own meanings for thoughts, actions, and events. In her mind, everything that happened to her, everything that touched her life, was caused by her. Correspondingly, she kept her own mind under constant observation, for if she could control what went on in her mind through her actions and thoughts, then she could control her life. If she translates all of the complexities of life into one problem—"I'm overweight"—then there is only one solution—"Lose weight."

All anorexics are obsessional, even those who weren't before they developed the disorder. Society accepts behavior that would otherwise be considered obsessional—preoccupation, over-intellectuality, perfectionism—in such people as competitive athletes, musicians, attorneys preparing for trial, artists, craftsmen, Wall Street traders. Our value system assigns worth to such commitment when the goal is fame and money. No one accuses the athlete training for the Olympics, the dancer or the ice skater who may practice obsessively, as being "sick." The efforts of these people relate to social goals with societally developed standards and limits.

A person has an obsessional disorder when his or her goal, the methods used toward obtaining that goal, and the constant repetition of those methods become one never-ending process and the pursuit has no finish line. A person has an obsessional disorder when the percentage of the individual's thinking and acting time dedicated to this pursuit is disproportionate to his or her time allotted for other aspects of daily life.

Because, in our society, the perceived rewards for a woman to become thin are so very high, thinking and acting to lose weight can become addictive. In this case, the difference between addiction and obsession is that most addictions involve substance abuse, which alters one's state of consciousness and whose usage and its effects have finite time limits. Rather than causing a pleasurable change in the way one experiences consciousness (as most addictive behavior does), obsessional behavior usually adds to the individual's anxiety level. Additionally, obsessional behavior is subject to infinite repetition because, as we saw, there is no "finish line." Whereas the addictive personality can get high enough or drunk enough, the obsessional personality will never "get there." There is no "fix" for an obsession.

So we see that while the pursuit to lose weight can be addictive, anorexia nervosa does not meet all of the criteria to qualify as an addiction. Then, considering the meaning of "compulsive" as defined in the "Security-Compulsive Stage" (see chapter 3), it is possible to classify anorexia nervosa as "an obsessional disorder with compulsive and addictive features."

The anorexic is obsessed with losing weight, becoming thinner.

Actions that produce weight loss feel like achievements. When the anorexic observes that she has lost weight, she experiences a sense of satisfaction but not completion; there is always more weight to be lost. In this vigilant pursuit, the anorexic continuously sees a need to lose weight in order to keep the obsession centered. Again we see where obsession differs from addiction. There is, at no point, even temporary satiety; any satisfaction is merely momentary.

This endless, insatiable pursuit ultimately molds the anorexic's identity: "fat-fighter." The human mind must identify its enemy before it can begin to fight it. In this case, the enemy is targeted as body fat. This is why anorexics see fat where there is none. That is what causes the famed distortion in self-perception of body image that is associated with anorexia.

Individuals who are unable to form attachments or trust others are emotionally incapable of receiving support, reassurance, or comfort from other people. For example, if I don't really know how to trust in other people, then how could I believe you if you told me I'm handsome or smart, or I've lost enough weight and now I can stop? In this vein, such a person is also incapable of allowing others to affect his or her judgment to limit his or her impulses and feelings when they become extreme, out of touch with reality. The replacement for reality, the *inner* reality with its conveniently complete solutions, is maintained with a ferocious intensity and desperation. It is as if the anorexic would lose all sense of mental organization if he or she was to give up this self-created system.

A person's ability to utilize the advice of others depends on very early childhood experiences with dependency, attachment, and trust. If these experiences are positive, the individual will not have to invent an alternate reality with an alternate version of what he or she experiences and internal, obsessive solutions for all problems. Positive early childhood experiences can successfully lead to a healthy attitude toward trust in relationships as well as the ability to communicate our needs in adulthood. However, a trauma in childhood, adolescence, or even adulthood will undermine that trust and cause it to disintegrate. The result: an obsessional withdrawal away from others and into oneself.

Trauma-induced withdrawal into the obsession of anorexia nervosa and the sense of safety and control it seems to provide can occur at almost any stage of life. It is, however, more likely to be a retreat for those younger than thirty.

Medical trauma, especially related to the throat or digestive system, has been the springboard for many cases of anorexia even where early childhood experiences were positive. Often in these instances the anorexic does have genetic tendencies toward anxiety that never proved problematic until the trauma occurred.

JOHN

John came to treatment at the age of twenty-four. He had developed anorexia; at six foot one, he was reduced to an emaciated one hundred and five pounds. He had no prior history of eating disorders. Four years before he walked into the office he had developed irritable bowel syndrome, along with duodenitis (the early deterioration of his stomach lining that would eventually lead to an ulcer). Because of these two afflictions, whatever food was good for John's stomach caused bowel inflammation, pain, and diarrhea. Conversely, whatever he ate that was good for his bowel hurt his stomach. John was in constant pain.

At some point, John lost faith in the medical and nutritional specialists he had turned to for help and began to withdraw from the people around him. He was afraid to eat anything for fear that the wrong choice would cause him one sort of physical distress or another. Reducing his eating in an effort to avoid the pain that plagued him caused extreme weight loss, which he ignored until others called it to his attention out of their concern for him. John reconciled himself to the idea that he was simply a thinner person than he had been. Becoming thinner had not been a goal for John, it was just how things turned out. This transformation occurred over a period of several months during which his digestive discomfort was greatly reduced, as was his consumption of food. As he slowly withdrew from the advice of others (advice that had failed to improve his original suffering), he also withdrew from his emotional attachments to people, preferring to avoid pain at all costs.

Loss of weight contributes to increased obsessionality and social withdrawal (Ansel Keys, 1950).[*] John found himself not only equating decreased eating with less pain, but also (by association) with weighing less. In his case, to gain weight meant to eat more; or, in its abbreviated logic, to gain weight meant to be in pain.

John was determined not to eat enough to gain weight, even though he understood that he was severely underweight. No health considerations, or the people who discussed them, mattered any more. Because of the mind's ability to abbreviate steps to a goal, skill, or action, John found himself believing that being thin meant being safe. Withdrawal into anorexia was a much safer path than heeding the failed promises of those he consulted about his health. John had developed "atypical" anorexia nervosa.

To understand the phenomenon of obsessiveness, we must first examine the person whose experiences led him or her to "break" all attachments, trust in, and dependency on others. Some people never develop this connection; some develop it and lose it due to overpowering events in their lives (as John did). If these individuals are girls or women, they are prone to succumb to the lure of obsessiveness over body weight. This is the most likely path for the female who has broken from trust relationships because our society suggests that being overweight is the worst way in which a woman can fail. Others yield to obsessiveness about contamination and become hand-washers, or are obsessive doubters who become checkers

[*]Ansel Keys and his associates published, in 1950, a definitive study on the biology of starvation, defining the psychological effects of human starvation and establishing their existence independent of neurosis and psychosis"—Sours (1980), p. 211. See Recommended Reading.

(checking and rechecking buttons, zippers, stove knobs, door locks, etc.). Sadly enough, some people fall victim to all of these obsessions. One can speculate that this was the case with Howard Hughes, but without taking a closer look it is mere conjecture.

In the processes of the human mind, "meaning" is the way the individual interprets personal experience and the actions, thoughts, and events that come with that experience. Once the mind utilizes a major idea for meaning, it continues to expand the usage of this mode of interpretation to include more and more of what it thinks about or processes. For example, if (because of a life experience or lack of trust-relationship development) I don't ever feel safe, I might translate a temporary feeling of social insecurity into wondering if my door is locked. Following the pattern just described, more and more of what I do, think, and feel would occur to me in the form of conscious worrying about whether my door was locked.

One way to revise this mode of thinking, which is called "obsessiveness," is to help the person reattach, re-depend on, retrust the people that he or she has either separated from or never sufficiently attached to in the first place. Such people are usually ones who were key figures in the person's young life, such as parents or siblings. The process of relationship detachment is necessary in order for obsessiveness to develop.

The pattern I outlined earlier that brought me from feeling socially insecure to obsessing about whether or not my door was locked, is a process I refer to as "abbreviation." Abbreviation is the way in which a person's mind teaches itself to move from step one directly to step eight because of learned patterns of thinking. Abbreviation occurs on both the mental and emotional levels.

A healthy example of abbreviation can be seen when one learns to drive a car. Initially, the new driver is bombarded by an overwhelming awareness of all the tasks involved in controlling the vehicle: steering it so that it remains centered on the road, alternately applying pressure to the brake pedal and the gas pedal in order to control the rate of velocity, being visually aware of the position and movement of other cars on the road, moving along the same road as the other cars without crashing into them, are all separate and very weighty mental considerations.

As the driver becomes more experienced, the mind coordinates the driver's movements with less and less conscious thought about what it's doing. Through learning by practice or repetition, the driver's mind *abbreviates* the thinking it originally did about each individual step. The experienced driver maneuvers the vehicle unselfconsciously.

Abbreviation allows us to learn new skills without cluttering our minds with the detailed steps of every skill that we learned in the past. Abbreviation is also what transfers thoughts of these now-unnecessary details to our mental filing system, the unconscious.

Anorexia nervosa includes a pathological or unhealthy use of abbreviation. During the first stage, the sufferer is merely eating less often for a justifiable purpose: to slim down to what the culture suggests is the correct physical appearance. The actions involved in slimming down (e.g., restricting calorie intake and fat consumption and increasing exercise) are all culturally dictated and nonobsessional in character and practice.

The crossover into pathological behavior occurs during stage two, the "Security-Compulsive Stage," when the dieter needs, or is compelled, to keep losing weight in order to relieve feelings of inadequacy, worry, anxiety, or other negative emotions.

At this point the individual is more intently monitoring the weight loss, metering it at usually around two pounds a week. During this stage, she begins to abbreviate from "I feel anxious so I'll eat less, lose weight, and feel better" to "I'm having a fat day." The sufferer skips over all the feelings and thoughts that are making her feel worried or upset, and, because of the practiced pattern mentioned above, immediately equates not feeling better with not having lost enough weight. Originally this person lost weight to feel better; now when she feels bad, it means with needing to lose weight—"feeling fat."

The abbreviated conclusion, "I feel fat," is the only thing that's left of all the complex worries, anxieties, and feelings, the thoughts of being a different dress size or looking more like the people on TV, that originally motivated the person to start losing weight. Because of this abbreviation that brought the victim automatically to convert any negative feelings into "feeling fat," this idea lingers long after it is realistic. Here we can see how the thin, emaciated anorexic who continues the effort to lose weight is victimizing him- or herself by an obsolete and pathological abbreviation of thoughts and feelings.

This substitution of fat feelings for all others allows anorexics to avoid confronting their emotions, and leaves all the real problems unsolved. After allowing unresolved problems to accumulate, the victim begins to use "fat ideas" more and more in order to "solve" everything. The only solution: losing weight. Of course, this brings the individual further and further from solving real problems as well as from relating to other people. Unconsciously, the anorexic begins to feel more in despair of coming back to any former reality, of resolving any of the real problems.

No one gambles more recklessly than the gambler who has lost the most. No one tries to succeed with less effort than the person who chronically feels in the poorest position. We call this state "despair." The more chronic the anorexia is, the more the victim has lost in terms of self-esteem, friendships, and hopes for future happiness. When this happens, the anorexic depends more deeply on her obsessive anorexic rules. At least she has those. She becomes little more than the sum of her anorexic characteristics.

Anorexia nervosa is unique among obsessional disorders because society invites girls and women to try to lose more weight than is healthy. Society supports launching these girls and women in the direction of a deprivation that will make sick those predisposed to its obsessional trap. Many times at parties women have made the joke, "You know, I wish I could get just a little of that anorexia." I always assure them that it only comes in one size—devastating.

5

THE PARENTS' ROLE IN PREVENTING ANOREXIA IN CHILDREN

Parents Today

TODAY'S parents are among the most hardworking group ever. Economic expectations and assumptions are a great part of the reason for this development. We assume that a certain size home, air conditioning, the highest quality of education for our children will save them. We race to seek the safest neighborhoods to live in, while we have few community resources to protect us. Most two-parent families struggle, with both of them working a full-time job to allay the fear of falling out of the middle class into oblivion, American poverty. These pressures take their toll on parents and deplete their emotional and nurturing resources. "Quality time" becomes harder to come by when both parents come home exhausted. Nannies, and day-care facilities, for those who can afford them, pick up some of the strain, but do little to enrich the relationships that children need. Medical and psychiatric care is spread thinner in the political pretense that more of the population will benefit.

As if these factors weren't enough, to diminish the security of growing children, girls and women are pressured to be unnaturally thin, below their genetic weight and below their fertility weight. This final demand can often break the back of one's mental health. Women's service magazines dream up new excuses weekly to defend the thinness required of the fashion industry. Hollywood follows their lead, whether it's "policy" or individual female actors trying to compete for a cultural sense of adequacy or superiority (after all, they suffer from the same sense of insecurity about weight as the general population of women does). Models and female actors become the Judas Goats who lead all women to hate their bodies.

The spate of modern "twentysomething" or older shows on television are replete with a language of intimacy that rarely exists in real life. Teenagers (as well as pre-teens) hear allusions to masturbation, genitals, and sex in general, and feel they need to be as comfortable as these actors are with this kind of communication, or else they label themselves as hopelessly behind. These shows are geared more to the "fortysomething" audiences, where they may be comical and entertaining. For every teen who is "up to speed" socially about such subjects, many girls are frightened and become nearly sexually despairing.

The thin models and actors probably have the same effect on the general population in terms of achieving the "right" weight. Their despair about being thin enough will cause them to give up the contest. Eventually, they become recklessly overweight in their hopelessness.

Clearly, many forces support or undermine the development of healthy families. But today there are fewer supportive elements, and the emphasis on undermining cultural factors, expectations of affluence, thinness, competition, and extreme independence all have their effects, especially on children and young adults. All of these factors also lower the self-esteem in parental identity, as they disenfranchise and compete with parents in establishing and maintaining sensible values for their children.

When are women emotionally capable of becoming nurturing, competent, limit-setting mothers? When do men become capable of being loving, warm, patient fathers? When do men and women become capable of becoming mutually supportive parents?

For some, the answer is never. For others, it is as early as when they become older sisters or older brothers. For others again, it is only when their children are fully grown. But for most people, this generational maturing occurs somewhere between the realization of pregnancy and the birth of the baby—"Whew, just in time."

Many women and men react differently to seeing themselves as parents. When my first child was born, I remember returning to our apartment excited and overwhelmed. I walked around the room reciting, "My daughter . . . Now *my* daughter . . . My *daughter*, on the other hand . . ." Her birth had profoundly changed my sense of identity. I was now a father, with added responsibilities that would affect my character and personality. I would never be the same again. But who would I become? What about my past—my childhood, my relationships with my brother, parents, my own sense of identity? How would these affect my "new" personality and the kind of parent I would become to my daughter? What kind of husband I would become to my wife?

When we want to understand a psychological disorder, we usually examine the hereditary-biological factors, the developmental-family factors, and the societal pressures affecting the individuals past and present.

Parental identity is not a psychological disorder, but it is part and parcel a result of the same factors, and one's reaction to them—the present functioning personality in a given circumstance. Parenting is rewarding, stressful, and demanding.

Every parent is someone's child. Every parent is subject to the same genetic, developmental, societal pressures, plus the responsibility for another person's development. The responsibility for another's development often brings out aspects of one's own personality and character that were unseen and not experienced before the birth of a child. The list includes following one's parents' model—"How they treated you is how you will treat your own children, compensating for unacceptable parental treatment"; or, "How they treated you is *never* how you'll treat your children"; or, the most complicated one, which I call *"My child feels like my parent."*

While some, consciously or unconsciously, copy parents' treatment they received as children and adolescents, others avoid anything that resembles their parents' treatment of them, making up to their child for the ways they had been wronged as children. For example, the child who was well behaved herself (perhaps resentfully) encourages rebelliousness in her child. The child who was given little affection and permissiveness gives his own child unending affection and permits the child to take charge of his own activities at a premature age.

These parenting profiles can been divided into three basic categories: the "imitative" parent; the "compensating" parent; and the "balanced" parent.

The Imitative Parent

Some parents, consciously or unconsciously, duplicate the treatment they received as children and adolescents in raising their own children. Every simple solution invites problems of its own. The imitative parent may find an ever-widening gulf between herself and her child as she applies culturally outdated rules to the child. Imitative parents may be courting rebellious or even delinquent behavior in their child.

Here is an example of imitative parents.

MEGAN

Megan was the daughter of two working-class parents. They were overworked and short-tempered. Her father drove a taxi and her mother worked for a dry cleaner. Often Megan would have to spend her afternoons in the back of the dry cleaning store where she was told to do her homework or "find some constructive way to keep busy." This routine began when she was three years old. She was scolded, glared at, and slapped by her mother, sometimes just for asking a question when her mother was busy with a customer. As she got older, she either assisted in the store or cooked dinner at home. Friends and playtime were nonexistent. When she grew up, Megan married a union electrician who earned enough money so they could buy their own modest home, and she worked part time.

When Megan gave birth to her daughter, Toni, she was annoyed with Toni's colic and occasionally spanked her out of frustration. Other times she would demand that her husband walk the floor with the baby until she stopped crying. Megan realized how much "trouble" her daughter was. Toni entered school, and would sometimes go to another child's house after school. She noticed that other children's mothers treated their children nicer. She adapted to her mother's negativity by becoming sneaky, lying to get away from her parents' house, stealing money from them, and eventually hanging out with kids who got into trouble using drugs and engaging in promiscuous sex. Toni also developed bulimia nervosa.

Megan felt betrayed by her daughter. She had given Toni a strict upbringing, the way she was raised by her own mother, yet Toni didn't comply with her mother's demands the way Megan had. So Megan felt angry and cheated. It seemed that the more pressure Megan put on her daughter, the greater the distance between them. Megan was, after all, behaving toward her daughter the way her mother behaved toward her. Why shouldn't she get the same cooperation her mother got from her?

Megan imitated her own mother's strict behavior. But unlike Megan, her daughter Toni sought refuge outside the family, in a peer group of other disaffected children. The peer group replaced their dependency on their parents with depending on each other. They used each other as co-conspirators in their rebellious behavior. Megan was puzzled and irritated by Toni's willfulness and defiance. She tried punishments; she grounded Toni, took her allowance away, listened in on Toni's phone calls, but all of these measures only made Toni more resourceful.

Megan wanted to defeat Toni's behavior because it would prove that she was a "good mother" in her own mother's terms. To add to Megan's stress, her own mother would telephone her to inquire about her grandaughter's behavior. Megan's mother was greeting her reports with disapproval, which reminded Megan of all the feelings of inadequacy she felt as a child. She was trapped between her mother's disapproval of her mothering and her daughter's rebelliousness.

Toni was only in her mid-teens and her rejection was not an indication of any real independence, maturity, or emotional self-sufficiency, but an ineffective way to show her mother that she needed something different from her.

But Megan had no other behavioral "tools" to deal with Toni. Megan had no other role models than her own mother. Surely, the cure for Toni was to "break her will" and return to the behavior her mother expected of her. Megan's husband believed that Toni was his wife's problem. That's how it was in his house, and even more so with a daughter. After all, how could a father know what a girl needed?

Megan was passively abandoned by everyone in her attempt to get support from her own mother and her husband. Her daughter seemed to abandon her as well.

Megan became depressed and rarely left the house except when she had to run an errand. Toni in turn became both frightened and angry at her mother's withdrawal. Somehow getting scolded was better than being ignored. She was alarmed that perhaps she actually had defeated her mother. One day her father commented to her in anger, "You know, kid, you're not the only member of this family who has problems." Toni became worried about her mother—something she didn't think she was capable of. She began to eat more, especially sweets, cakes, and doughnuts. She began to gain weight. Her friends teased her about looking fat. She began to vomit after eating, to avoid gaining weight.

If she went to a restaurant with her friends, she would check out the ladies' room to see if there was enough privacy to vomit undetected. She noticed that the drive to eat was becoming greater, the amounts she ate larger. Toni's vomiting became increasingly important. Securing a "safe" place to vomit became a preoccupation for her. It somehow played into the feelings she got from tricking her mother to sabotage her mother's attempt to punish her. After awhile Toni couldn't tell which was more gratifying: eating large quantities of food, vomiting, or the "adventure" of finding a sneaky way to vomit undetected. She was well entrenched in the vomiting when it became apparent to her that she could not only prevent herself from gaining weight but she could use the vomiting to lose weight, maybe even become the thinnest of her friends.

Toni had remained adept at vomiting undetected, but when she began to lose weight, it was noticeable. At first, her friends complimented her on the initial ten pounds she lost. After that, the compliments ceased until she began to be criticized for "going too far" and looking too thin. Toni smiled to herself when the new criticism by her friends intensified. Her parents were still focused on her general rebelliousness, which in fact had diminished as Toni became more involved in losing weight.

Toni had lost twenty-five pounds before her parents noticed. Even after they remarked to each other about her weight loss, they concluded it was less troublesome than her rebellious attitude had been. They let the subject go until Toni had lost another ten pounds. At that time she was five foot four and weighed ninety-nine pounds. A friend of hers called her mother during the school day knowing that Toni wouldn't be at home. The friend informed Megan that the school nurse had sent Toni to the school guidance counselor to explore the possibility that she was developing anorexia and that the counselor would be calling home shortly. Toni had told her friend all this, somewhat alarmed.

Megan had never thought that her daughter cared what anyone thought about what she did. She was surprised at her own reaction to the friend's call. After thanking the friend for calling, she sat down on a kitchen chair and pondered her daughter's alarm. For the first time in quite a while her anger toward her daughter melted into sympathy and worry. Her worry increased when she remembered that she had little control or influence over her daughter's behavior. If she *was* developing anorexia, what could Megan do to stop the weight losing? She knew how deceptive her daughter could be over any issue. That's when she decided to seek professional help.

The Compensating Parent

Compensating parents will avoid anything that resembles their own parents' approach to raising them as children. Thus, they will make up to the child for the way they themselves were wronged as children. For example, the child who was well behaved, and perhaps resented that, encourages rebelliousness in her child. The child who was given little affection and permissiveness gives her own child unending affection and permits the child to be in charge of her own activities at a premature age.

The compensating parent may find that the child becomes tyrannical and the parent becomes the resentful servant of a child who has no boundaries. The problem here is that the parent is unconsciously compensating the "wronged" child, the parent, by spoiling his or her own child, who was never wronged.

It is the compensating parent who is likely to find herself (himself) "wronged" by her own child in the same way she feels wronged by her own parents. I call this "the my parents, myself," bind, because it puts the parent in the same unsatisfactory position with her parents as with her child.

Compensating parents may be inadvertently developing mistrust and obsessiveness in their child.

Here is a case study of a compensating parent.

ALBA

Alba was brought up in Costa Rica. Her parents were strict. Her father ruled her mother, but her mother ruled Alba with laws, mandates, and regulations about everything from the way she dressed, spoke, stood, and ate, to how she played with her friends. Her mother even chose her friends.

When Alba graduated from the university, she left for the United States. She went into banking and married a co-worker. Alba desperately wanted to have a daughter. She was sure she knew how to raise a child. She would give her everything her mother never gave her: choices, permission, praise, affection, even deference. Amy, her daughter, developed into an independent child, highly successful in school, with lots of friends. But Amy was difficult and moody at home. At times Amy felt like the tyrant Alba's mother was. Nevertheless, Amy was successful in so many ways that Alba felt she didn't have the right to criticize her. Alba believed that she had avoided all the mistakes her mother had made with her. She did everything in the opposite way her mother did in raising her daughter. She never made her daughter feel all the hurt her mother made her feel. She supported her daughter in all the ways her mother failed to support her. She compensated her daughter for all the grievances she had suffered as a child at her mother's hands. The problem here was that Amy was not Alba! Alba was making it up to *herself*, confusing herself and her own needs with Amy's. She had compensated the wrong victim. Amy developed anorexia nervosa at the age of fifteen.

When Amy turned fifteen, she developed a crush on a boy in her class. She didn't know how to attract his attention and grumbled to herself, "It's too bad that there's no course in this school on flirting." She smiled at him, bumped into him, asked him about the homework assignment, but he just rushed off after politely answering her question. She didn't know what to do.

One evening she was staring in the mirror, trying to decide what to wear the next day. First, she looked through the clothes in her closet, then she decided to consult her fashion magazines. She began with the two most popular that pre-teen girls read, but quickly moved on to the women's magazines. She leafed through looking for articles containing hints on "How to catch that man who doesn't know you're alive." The more she studied the magazines, the more she examined the figures of the models. As she took stock, she made mental notes: "their legs are unbelievably long, they must be very tall." She noticed that in many cases the models' statistics were included in the layout. "Five eleven! No wonder. I don't understand how they can be that thin and have such big boobs. When I lose weight, mine get smaller! That's the first place I lose weight. It can't be exercise."

Amy walked over to the mirror. She stood as straight and tall as she could. She put on her highest-heeled shoes. "Hmm, a little better," she thought. She stretched her chest muscles to make her stick out as far as possible. Her breasts still looked small. Her limbs didn't look long enough. She wet her lips and pursed them in the mirror. "Full enough," she thought. "Well, if I can't make my legs longer, I can make them thinner so they'll look longer. Then he'll notice me. I'll wear short, elastic skirts. Boys always stare at the hemline to see how far up they can see. Then he'll notice me," she repeated aloud.

Just then there was a knock at the door—a soft, tentative knock. "It's her," she thought contemptuously. "Come in." Her voice reflected her contempt for her mother. Amy forgot she was wearing only her underwear and high heels. Her mother was surprised and shocked by her daughter's appearance. Amy had lost ten pounds, but she was thin to begin with: at five six, one hundred and five pounds. Now at ninety-five pounds she was more than thin. To her mother, she looked emaciated.

"Well? What are you staring at?"

Her mother, characteristically timid, especially when her daughter used that annoyed tone, answered with a question: "Have you lost weight? You look terribly thin."

"If you look at my fashion magazines, you'll see I don't look any thinner than those models. You'll always be a worrier. I'm just getting in style is all." Amy's tone was so dismissive, her mother could barely muster an expression of disapproval as she walked out the door. She felt frightened and helpless, needing time to think of a strategy to cope with this new and terrifying problem.

The Balanced Parent

The third category is achieved by balance on the part of parents. This group falls into neither trap one nor trap two. Balanced parents maintain a combination of warmth, support, sensitivity, and awareness of their child's needs. They are not sending frightened or needy messages to their child, and they set appropriate limits when they feel that their child is making a mistake. It is clear that this category is the most rewarding for both parent and child—a difficult balance to achieve, but well worth pursuing. Children of balanced parents are not predisposed to eating disorders.

Parents can work toward greater balance by focusing on their child's needs and exhibiting the following behaviors:

1. *Warmth and calm* in the face of provocative behavior like skipping a meal or bingeing.
2. *Authority*—taking the lead, setting limits, and making rules.
3. *Self-confidence*—exhibited by optimistic behavior and talking in an even tone; offering reassurances and positive statements despite the child's expressions of despair and hopelessness.
4. *Communication*—especially important with difficult issues, despite your child's efforts to turn you away or reject your input. Remember that *communication* with your child is not the same as *controlling* your child.

Modifying Parental Identity

Finally, when a child is ill, we may have to *modify* our techniques of parenting. The changing course of her development requires that we set down recommended principles of parental behavior that will succeed.

If it becomes difficult to modify parental behavior, then we have to analyze the origins of our own parental identity in order to understand what feelings of guilt, anger, esteem, and so on are present in danger. After these are fully understood, parents are freer to make changes without experiencing anxiety or resentment toward their child.

Anorexia was once a rare, or rarely reported, disorder. For the past twenty years, it has assumed epidemic proportions and shows no signs of quitting. We will assume at this point that heredity affecting the biochemistry of depression and anxiety has not changed. Therefore, we must try to understand how economic and social pressures, as well as societal changes, influence the incidence of this disorder.

6

THE FAMILY SYSTEM AND THE ROLE
OF THE ANOREXIC CHILD

FAMILY changes when one of its members courts starvation, and these changes usually follow a pattern. When the diagnosis is first made, the family becomes anxious, worried, and often alarmed. These are normal reactions when a family has been told that a member has developed a serious, possibly chronic, sometimes even fatal disease: self-starvation.

The family has a difficult time believing that their daughter (or son) is involved in such unreasonable, irrational, "crazy" behavior. Anger is interwoven with fear. Often parents and siblings find themselves on an emotional roller coaster of fear–anger–guilt toward the sufferer. The only topics dominating family discussions with their anorexic child relate to food and exercise. Often other members of the family try to eat more to "encourage" the anorexic member to eat. Sometimes the entire family, especially the mother, gains weight in order to coax weight on the afflicted.

Ultimately, the family discovers that these strategies have failed and the afflicted member has become a source of anger for all its members. As she continues to lose weight, the family discovers that their anger is as ineffective as their "caring" strategies have been. They become polarized, divided, as each member rides the roller coaster. Suddenly the family seems hopelessly divided; everyone disagrees with everyone else. Gloom settles over the entire household.

Ironically, the most powerful member of the family becomes the anorexic herself. Her power is the change in her eating habits. This is her weapon. "I can't eat if you're in the kitchen," she declares, and everyone leaves the kitchen. "I can't eat if you're in the next room," and everyone leaves the next room. "I can't eat if you're in the house," and everyone goes to the garage while she eats. Absurd? Perhaps, but it comes close to that in this terrible power shift in the family system.

MYRA

Myra started to lose weight during her freshman year at college. Her three roommates didn't think Myra was overweight. They told her so. When she began to look pale and emaciated, they talked to her in an attempt to stop her pursuing thinness. They gave up in frustration and reported their observations to the dean. She sent for Myra and was alarmed that Myra had become emaciated "under everyone's nose." The dean referred Myra to Student Services, who in turn referred her to Medical Services to make sure that her thinness wasn't caused by diabetes, cancer, or other medical reasons. When all of Myra's tests came back negative, she was diagnosed by Student Services as having anorexia nervosa. The school notified her parents. Myra was assigned a counselor who was familiar with eating disorders and told Myra that at some point she would be asked to leave school if she continued to lose weight. She now weighed ninety-eight pounds.

Her parents were shocked when they arrived at her school and saw their five-foot-six daughter, who had left home at a hundred and twenty pounds, looking pale, her hair thinning. They had seen her last eight weeks earlier. The notice about her deteriorating health coincided with Parents' Weekend, an event they had anticipated with joy.

The drive home from college provoked intense confrontation. Myra alternately ranted and raved about how unfair the college had been in suspending her until she gained weight, and burst into tears. Her parents listened passively for the first two hours, trying to see their daughter's side and put aside her emaciated appearance. Myra sat in the backseat. Both parents, who were in the front seats, avoided turning around while talking to her.

After two hours, her father interrupted one of Myra's tirades by saying, "I guess the dean's position is that the college resigned as your guardian because they felt helpless to stop you from losing weight."

"Bullshit!" Myra retorted. "There are skinnier kids than me on campus and no one is throwing them out!"

At that point Myra's father, stopped at a traffic light, turned around, glared at her, and shouted, "Do you know what you look like? *Do you know what you have done to yourself?*"

Myra burst into tears again. "I don't know why everyone is picking on me. So I lost a little weight, what's the big deal? Is that a reason to throw me out of college? What good is that going to do?"

Myra's father was stopped by her logic on the narrower issue of the school's policy for a moment, but recovered by remembering the larger issue. "The school's decision to 'throw you out,' as you put it, is a result of this drastic and . . . yes, *crazy* thing that you've done to yourself. Have your roommates and friends mentioned that your appearance is bizarre, or do they think you look normal?"

Silence.

"Well," he repeated, "what have other students said to you about your appearance?"

"They said I look too thin," she said unwillingly.

"Do you understand how serious this is? You have been asked to leave school. Your friends think that you look too thin, and you look to me as if you're on your way to starving to death. Does that strike you as strange?"

"I don't think that I'm so thin," Myra said meekly.

"I think you're lying. I think that you know how serious this is and that you're too ashamed to admit it."

Myra's mother remained quiet throughout this confrontation. She was afraid that her husband was talking too harshly to her daughter and that his harshness might make her "sicker." Now she tried to mediate what sounded like an argument to her. "Peter, we have plenty of time to talk about this at home. We have a problem, or rather, Myra has a problem, and I think that we'll need professional help for her."

Myra cut her off. "What's with this 'professional help' business? I saw a counselor at Student Services and she didn't make me feel any different. What's somebody else going to do?"

Silence. No one knew what to do and Myra's comments succeeded in making everyone feel helpless. Myra's anorexia won.

Usually parents are present when the insidious weight loss behavior starts. There is a vague area where parents don't know whether their intervention is needed or not. The victim herself may not be aware when she becomes *compelled* to lose the weight and the goal of losing a number of pounds no longer exists. She, as well as her parents, may not be able to determine when weight loss becomes an illness. By this time, the daughter has undergone a period of weight loss without anyone's objection. She will not tolerate a change in their attitude now.

Parents have a hard time shifting gears from acceptance to objection to their daughter's dieting. In Myra's case, it was an easy call. The long car ride from her college to her home, coupled with the school psychologist's diagnosis, compressed the beginning of the struggle between Myra and her parents. Myra used denial to defend her disease. Her parents, armed with the shock of seeing her "sudden" change along with the school's definitive statement that she had anorexia nervosa, tried to confront her with the reality of her situation. But her parents' fear, anger, and guilt were ineffective against Myra's defiant tears and depression.

A strategy that would change these patterns requires a reevaluation of family relationships, individual psychotherapy for Myra, and family therapy or couples' therapy for her parents.

How the Family System Is Affected by the Disorder

In a typical family, this is how members respond to anorexia:

The mother is usually immobilized, guilty, frightened, and will later become angry at her daughter, but reverts to all other states when anger is spent, or acted upon.

The father is typically confused, resentful, mystified, feels sorry for himself, worried for his daughter.

The daughter is enraged, defending her anorexic behavior (restrictive eating, over-exercising) when confronted by her parents. Fiercely independent and dependent at the same time, she is secretly ashamed of herself. Away from the family, she is easily intimidated by others if the issue is not about her eating and weight. She will defer to others about what movie to see, what friends to include.

Siblings are angry, frustrated, mystified, disappointed in their anorexic sister. They are also unconsciously afraid that their sister's illness will take parental attention away from them as their sister becomes the focus of the family. They may become abusive to their sister as a result of this fear, which will quickly turn into jealousy. They may attempt to prove to the parents that *they* are the *best* children, and the parents should not "spoil" their sister for being "stubborn" about her eating and weight.

Parents are faced with a double dilemma:

1. How strict or permissive should they be with their anorexic daughter in supervising her eating and exercising? Should they "butt in" or "butt out"?
2. How do they deal with other siblings when they receive complaints about either strategy? They also need to take a consistent posture with the other children and should assign them a role in terms of their sister. The parents have the additional

burden of balancing their attention to other children while focusing on their anorexic child.

Clearly, these complex issues place enormous demands on parents. If there is only one parent, the demand is doubled, and the single parent will definitely need his or her own support system, whether from parents, friends, clergypeople, or psychological professionals. Of course, the same need for additional support is necessary for two parents coping with this problem.

Reorganizing the Family System

The first priority for a family handling an anorexic child is unity and mutual support. If there are two parents in the family system, their first task is to compare their views on the afflicted child. Are they polarized? Does one parent think that he or she has to protect the child from the other? Does the other parent think that the child is being overprotected, or "babied" by the first parent?

If parents are at odds, we have a contest between them that is dangerously divisive. Parents will be suspicious of each other, undermine each other, and convince the child that neither parent knows what they are doing. This parental tension provides no security to the child. The child then invents her own set of ideas and rules to replace both parents. Since she knows that her rules have been invented by a child (adolescent), they have to be over-observed to compensate for the dubiousness of their source. This over-observation becomes over-thinking, which in turn becomes obsession. All anorexics are obsessive in that they over-think their weight-control behavior. Obsessive people tend to be rigid, fearing that flexibility will result in mental chaos.

Creating a Parental Team

The first task in creating a solid, effective parent team is letting go of our own ego and identity. We don't parent from our soul, no matter how much we love our children. Parenting is a combination of aptitude and style, based on one's own parental role models. All of these elements are up for revision without condemning the parent for revising his or her style. When parents reparent their anorexic child, they must do so *with one voice*. This important aspect of change requires a lot of parental communication without the child's presence. Parents should resolve their differences in private and offer advice or set limits together. For example, their daughter may want to continue dance classes although she is not yet regaining her weight. By discussing the decision first, her parents have the opportunity to judge the pros and cons of this activity without arguing in front of her.

If the anorexic is being parented by divorced parents, they must put aside their own differences in the interest of *competing with the anorexia*. It is important to remember that anorexia becomes an entity, a strong voice in the victim's mind. Parents and therapists are the only ones who have the moral power to compete with this voice, to lure her away from it, toward health.

If the anorexic is being parented by a single parent, she (or he) will need an additional support system to help change the style of their relationship. This is an enormous undertaking, and outside help is vital. The poor recovery rate (about 25–35 percent) can be attributed to the underestimation of how much energy and effort are required on the part of caretakers—parents, therapists, even hospitals.

The most important concept to bear in mind on the part of parents, therapists, and others is that the anorexic is *mentally ill*. This may sound harsh, but it will aid the parents and other helpers in maintaining ego distance so that they are not seduced or provoked, or made to feel guilty by this powerful mind-set that dominates its victim.

Considering one's child mentally ill does not mean that everything she says should be ignored or that she should be patronized. Instead, parents need to hear her words as an expression of the disease. All her talk about weight, eating, exercise, and elimination is prompted by the disease. When her parents respond reasonably about nutritional and medical reality, this becomes provocative and challenging to her anorexic belief system and invites rage, tears, or sulking. Reacting to these feelings may be difficult for some families, especially if they have avoided arguments in the past. The purpose is not to produce arguments and conflicts, but to confront them when raised, and to let their daughter know that her family's resolve is stronger than her anorexic ideas and that their strength is more attractive than the anorexic tyrant that lives within her. If the family is drawn into arguing about eating portions, exercise, and so on, and gives in to these arguments, then the family is inadvertently giving a message to the anorexic that her ideas have validity.

An anorexic is emotionally closer to her disease than she is to her family. Our goal is to transfer that balance so that the anorexic is more allied with her family, and the disease is the common enemy. The same is true for the therapist. We need to change all balances of alliance so that the victim is fighting her disease along with those who are helping her.

While seeming to be genuinely outgoing, the anorexic has, for the most part, "kept her own counsel," not really depending upon anyone else to help her feel more secure. This is especially true when the source of her insecurity lies with her if she has feelings of insecurity, anxiety, or poor self-esteem, but can't trace these feelings to a specific external cause, such as doing poorly on a test in school or not being invited to a party.

In order to balance the family system, parents will need to be aggressive in encouraging their overly independent or hostile-dependent daughter to trust them with her eating, weight, and exercise, and to trust their judgment. Here there is no room for equivocation or uncertainty in one's response to a decision that has to be made in a dispute between parent and daughter. This is not to be construed as unfair or harsh treatment. Instead, it should be seen as a firm response, warmly stated.

"Mom, I can't eat this chicken, it's too fattening."

"It's not fattening and you need the nutrition to gain weight. I know you're scared but you have to try to gain weight, even though it's so hard for you."

To look at this concept from an anorexic's point of view, her question is, "Is the voice in my head that tells me not to eat stronger than the voices of those around me?" Will she reward parents who follow this advice? Absolutely not. She will fight back, resist, try to make the parents feel guilty. Anorexia does not give up without a fight.

The struggle could last for months. This period of resistance is the "testing" period, the time needed to make tentative trust jell into positive attachment and healthy dependency. The stress of the struggle may turn parent against parent, other siblings against the anorexic sibling as well as the parents. The illness brings family divisiveness no matter how it is handled. We will have to term this period of testing, where the disease is attacking the family system, "productive conflict" as opposed to random divisiveness.

Heartbreak, Denial, and Chaos in the Family System

It is far easier to hide mental illness in the family than physical illness. For hours or even days at a time, parents can avoid awareness of mental illness, especially if their child makes reasonable statements much of the time, as is the case in anorexia, anxiety disorders, phobias, bulimia, even episodic depression, to name but a few. There is an unconscious wish on the part of parents that the illness should be part of normal adolescence, impatience, stubbornness, even brattiness. Medically, this kind of wish is termed *denial*. Denial functions to disguise the heartbreak, fear, and despair the family experiences when the illness is diagnosed, or "out in the open." This denial elevates parents' expectations of their child to those for a "normal" child. It turns their sadness about their child into annoyance, anger, and rage. Such feelings are easier to tolerate but don't foster recovery; rather, they create chaos and divisiveness between members of the family. These feelings also confuse the identified patient, causing her to withdraw more deeply into her illness for protection. Her withdrawal may then cause the family to be more angry at her as the cycle of chaos accelerates.

When this occurs, usually an outside professional needs to be brought in as a referee/interpreter for the family. This provides some distance from the immediate conflict for each member of the family so that the problem can be put in proper perspective. "Neglected" siblings, even a neglected spouse, may have to express their feelings during a family therapy session. When one member of the family becomes ill, the rest of the family can hardly be expected to become saints in response. If any change at all is to happen, it will be along the lines of a drain of nurturance affecting all members of the family.

Parents don't want to believe that they have a mentally ill child; younger siblings don't want to believe that their older sibling, who they need to look up to, is "defective." Older siblings often develop a sense of guilt about their younger sibling. Maybe they neglected her, excluded her, or bullied her too much. The heartbreak and disappointment usually affects everyone. When the heartbreak is unbearable, denial replaces it with "normal" expectations and anger directed toward the mentally ill member of the family. In the case of the anorexic, this usually takes the form of "You are lying about what you eat." Punishment is often used, further separating the nontrusting anorexic from those around her. Tempers flare, tears are shed. Despair takes over. "Stubborn, crazy kid" replaces "lost, sick kid" in the minds, feelings, and conversations of family members. If this reaction is not mediated, it becomes the chronic cycle of the family system which produces chronic anorexia, as well as other chronic psychiatric disorders.

An anorexic child in the family is under the influence of a psychological, or psychiatric, disorder. We have to understand that she is out of reach in terms of seeing things and reacting to situations the way the rest of us do. Failing to remember the out-of-reach part separates us further from our common context, disappoints us, makes us angry and frustrated with the anorexic, and makes her recovery less likely.

As the pressure on the family to simultaneously love their daughter and maintain a perspective on her illness increases, it is also necessary not to take her insulting and aggressive behavior personally. The reason most families turn to psychotherapists for both individual and family therapy is the overwhelming nature of the demands for patience, understanding, and "correct" behavior that the illness places on them. They need support, supervision, understanding, interpretation, and advice on a continuing basis. To combat this illness, the family will need enormous psychological energy and commitment.

7

THE SOCIAL ORIGINS OF FEMININITY

KIM

IM'S father was a lawyer. He had been a scholarship student at one of the country's finest law schools. He was her hero, her ideal. Unfortunately, his highly successful career required that he work seventy to eighty hours a week, even though he was a full partner in a prominent law firm. Kim often saw her father at public events, where he was the center of attention.

Kim's mother was an even-tempered, calm, intelligent woman who stayed at home full time to raise her five children and manage their affluent house. She had one housekeeper to help. Kim's mother remained in the background, steadily taking care of her child and her husband. Kim respected her and was intimidated when she displeased her mother. When I asked Kim to discuss her mother, she would invariably get two sentences into the subject and suddenly change to talking about her father.

Kim came to therapy with a diagnosis of anorexia. She was "suspiciously" thin in appearance, though not frighteningly so. She was nineteen years old, five foot six, and weighed one hundred pounds.

Kim's mother described her as the ideal child. "She never needed supervision. She did well in school, with friends, and at home she was like a little mother to her younger sister [four years younger]. She was always concerned with everyone's well-being. She was a pure delight." Kim's mother explained that Kim had had a bout with anorexia at the age of twelve. It lasted about eight months, never so severe that she needed hospitalization. She was treated by a child psychiatrist whom she liked. When she recovered her weight and went on to high school, she kept her weight low, on that thin line between slender and "suspicious." This kept her parents on guard for four years, never knowing if and when the anorexia would recur.

When she left for college, they were worried but did not voice it. Kim returned at Thanksgiving having lost seven pounds. Her weight had dropped from a hundred and nine to a hundred and two. Both parents protested, her mother more intensely than her father. Kim retorted by reminding them they had worried about her all through high school and nothing happened. She dismissed them as "overreacting" to a normal fluctuation in weight. They backed down at her scolding. After all, with the exception of her anorexia at twelve, she had always demonstrated competence in everything she did.

This idea made some tentative sense to them. They also didn't want to believe that Kim was sick again. At this time in her life it would mean that she would have to leave the excellent college she had gotten into. They were all so proud of her when the acceptance letter arrived in the mail. Her mother brought in the envelope with the letterhead on top. When Kim saw the thick envelope, she screamed out in delight: "I made it! The large envelope has all the forms for registration, course schedules, and other materials. The thin envelope is a short, polite letter of rejection!" She tore open the large envelope and screamed again, "Yes! I made it!" They were proud of her and of course shared the good news with members of the family and friends. She was their oldest child, their first to be accepted by a first-class college.

When Kim returned on Christmas break, she had lost another

seven pounds and weighed a ragged ninety-five pounds. Her parents were both enraged. They had been tricked. Kim was told that she could not return to college for the winter term unless she gained ten pounds in the next six weeks. Kim was tearful and tried to protest that they were overreacting, but her protests fell on deaf ears and she knew it. She spent much of her day in her room. Her parents suspected that she was secretly exercising behind her closed door. What was surprising to them were the phone calls from boys she had met in college. When her mother asked about her popularity, glad for a chance to talk to her about anything other than her weight and appearance, Kim replied that some were "friends," and she didn't care about the ones who were romantically interested. Her mother was surprised at her indifference to these boys. She decided to question Kim, in session, at my office.

"Dear, don't you have any interest in boys? I know you didn't date in high school, but I chalked it up to your perfectionism about grades, and that paid off." Her mother tried to sound positive and enthusiastic, but she was offering her daughter an opportunity to express the possibility that she was a lesbian. Her daughter missed none of this. With a bitter, contemptuous frown, she responded dryly, "No, Mother, I'm not a lesbian. I'm . . . nothing. I mean, I'm nothing sexually. I just don't care about it—or boys."

"But you're so pretty, you always have been, everybody has always commented on it—not just to me or your father, but to you!" Her mother was saddened by what her daughter was telling her.

"Well, I never *felt* it. It never felt real. I thought that you all were just being nice. And when you say it . . . well, I'm your daughter. What else would you say? Daddy almost never says it and when he does, it always sounds so forced, so phony. Maybe he's the most honest." She stared at the floor, looking defeated. Her father was not present at this exchange.

I inquired, "Do you ever find a boy attractive?"

She looked up from the floor as if she'd forgotten I was there. "Yes, I think some boys are attractive, but I don't think that it matters."

"Why doesn't it matter?" I probed.

"Because it doesn't matter. Nothing could possibly come of it. So I stopped noticing boys or caring about them or hoping about them."

"Your mother says they must have been noticing you since they've been calling you all the time you've been home. It's been six weeks. That's a long time to receive continuous calls from boys you don't see because none of you are on campus for this break."

"I don't know how to answer you because it just doesn't seem to matter to me at all. I don't know why, it just doesn't."

"Let me just ask you a question. How do you feel about your father?"

"My father? Well, I guess what I feel about my father is . . . the same as I feel about all the other guys."

Kim was expressing a depressed sense of femininity, of desirability, of lack of interest in the opposite sex. Some of that is a function of low weight, which causes a decrease in hormone production, but it was obvious that Kim had little interest in boys, except as friends, even when her weight was normal. Her complaint about her father was a protest.

A Sense of Femininity

With all the strides women have made in the work place, one wonders why they have to strive too for the "perfect" appearance from head to toe. So many women seem to spend time and money pursuing a "perfect" appearance; diet, exercise, and plastic surgery are just a part of this frenetic pursuit. What is the "best" appearance a woman can achieve? And why such intensity (or despair) about it?

The male ego, in terms of pursuing women, is quite fragile. If a man doesn't see a woman as desirable visually, he doesn't respond sexually. It would then be healthy for women to seek ways to be seen as sexually desirable, in order to stir up that male libido in a manner that would preserve the species. Ironically, as society becomes more androgynous, men's libido diminishes for lack of defined roles and rules of restraint. As women become more assertive, that frail male libido shrivels up.

When women become less valued by men, and femininity becomes less valued by women, the competition among women for the best, superior body replaces the competition for attracting men. The original drive for seductive femininity for mating purposes has been twisted by societal elements into a feminine drive for unfeminine physical superiority among women, leaving seduction—and men—out of the picture. The drive for "physical success," even in its new, twisted form, bony or muscular, still retains the power and energy of nature's drive for seductive femininity.

Who does the twisting of this drive and why? The first observable changes in the "ideal" figure for women came in the early 1950s, when leading fashion magazines introduced dramatically thin models from France. They were often light-skinned, dark hair pulled back to add drama to their appearance. Women frequently either disapproved of this ideal figure or treated it comically, as when "Twiggy" was imported from England. But the new, dramatically thin models were here to stay. Women stopped deriding them and began to feel an urge to change their own appearance in the direction of the thin models relentlessly appearing monthly in the so-called women's service magazines. Interestingly enough, anorexia has always been with us in small numbers—a very rare disease indeed until the early seventies, it then began to assume epidemic proportions in Great Britain, the United States (one out of every two hundred and fifty), Canada, and now Japan. It has not diminished the way hairstyles or popular clothing designs have changed. Nor have the overly thin models left the women's magazine pages.

When the "waif look" reared its even skinnier head in the fall of 1994, women were finally incensed, and the fashion industry backed down by Christmas. Nobody in the industry talked "waif" any more. Still, the overly thin models persist, as does the fashion industry in dreaming up new reasons to explain why they prefer a boyish body in women's clothes. The effect of this phenomenon upon women helps to create eating disorders. It causes most women to hate their bodies — not because they are unattractive to men but because they are losing in the intense competition among women for a usually unattainable, unhealthy, thin body. Those who are thrown into despair about achieving this goal may go the other way to become part of the psychological subculture of obese women and compulsive overeaters.

Nearly all young girls and women are exposed to similar cultural messages and most do not develop anorexia or other eating disorders. Clearly, fashion and other pop culture media (including Hollywood's underweight actresses) are only part of the picture of what undermines physical femininity.

Where do girls get their earliest sense of femininity? This sort of question has all the risks of the "nature-nurture" controversy. Does the role-modeling of a mother, aunt, grandmother, or older sister provide the foundation upon which the young girl can behave and feel feminine? Perhaps "behavior" (dress, manners, etc.) might be distinguished from "feeling" feminine. Most girls assume that they will grow into women approximately like their mothers. If their mothers seem satisfied with their position in life, these girls become optimists about themselves and their futures. If their mothers seem dissatisfied, oppressed, abused, neglected, or depressed, the daughters are not looking forward to growing up and filling these undesirable roles. These girls may choose to identify with their fathers, who are doing better than their mothers.

If girls are supported by their parents, they develop confidence in themselves. If they identify with their mother's success, pursuit of their own success will be less conflict-ridden than if they have to identify with their fathers. If the latter is true, they will have to forego some of their sense of femininity in order to succeed in "masculine style."

Children whose parents do not act as cultural mediators, even cultural censors, are vulnerable to the hyperbolic messages of everything from the extremes of rap and rock music to violence on TV and in the movies. Parents' power to mediate negative, foolish, and even dangerous cultural messages depends on the trust, attachment, and dependency they have encouraged and received from their children. The societally "ideal" shape for women is one of these issues.

Fathers play an enormously important role in helping their daughters to feel feminine and to value that femininity. The "healthy" (as opposed to sexually exploitative) romance between father and daughter teaches little girls that it pays to be the apple of Daddy's eye. Verbal praise and appropriate physical affection provide feelings of feminine adequacy that can last a lifetime. Disengaged fathers, workaholic fathers, "busy" fathers who have no time to provide feminine support for their daughters, leave them with a blank neuter space where their feminine pride should be.

The absence of this pride is the absence of self-esteem. During their early teens and well before that, most girls experiment with their femininity; makeup, dress, posing in the mirror, are all preparatory steps for the time when they will really want to attract boys. At that time, they will have to have some self-confidence to dare to hope and to act on that hope that a particular boy may find them attractive. If they have a low sense of their feminine value or attractiveness, their feminine drives will lead them in other directions. Many of these directions will turn out to be unhealthy. One of them may be anorexia nervosa.

Like many other psychological disorders, anorexia is ultimately antisocial. The individual turns inward to a sealed system of perceived security that excludes the impact of others. Usually these systems—whether anorexia, obsessive-compulsive disorder, or phobia—increase in intensity until they take over the individual's life and most of her thinking, as well as behavior. She is more influenced by the ideas of her disorder than by her connection to others around her, no matter how much they care about her. She becomes, in effect, unreachable.

In earlier chapters, we saw the value of trust, attachment, and dependency. Now all these factors come into play. If there is significant trust, attachment, and dependency, and adequate father's input of feminine self-esteem, the likelihood of a girl drifting into "trusting" the messages of a disorder fostered by society is minimal. A girl who trusts her parents begins a diet and starts to become too thin. When she is told by one or both of her trusted parents, "That's enough weight loss, honey, you're looking too thin," she abides by their decision with a response like, "You really think so?" and she stops losing weight. The girl who has never had that bond simply dismisses her parents with a shrug and continues to lose weight. What they say to her has no impact, except perhaps an oppositional one, where she says to herself, "That's what you think." She keeps losing weight. And in the process, she compromises the physical and endocrinological aspects of her femininity.

8

BIOLOGICAL INFLUENCES

W HY are some children tense from birth? Children from the same family are often temperamentally different from one another. This can be observed in the delivery room, during infancy, in the toddler stage, and through puberty, even before the beginning of that destabilizing adolescent period. What do we know about the causes of these differences? How can therapists and parents compensate children who display excessive levels of anxiety? Identifying these problems early may avoid the development of psychological disorders such as anorexia nervosa, obsessiveness, and phobias. Even though some anxiety and depression is hereditary or biological, a therapeutic family system (and sometimes medication) can prevent these traits from evolving into complex disorders.

The medical debate over the chemical origins of depression will continue for some time to come. Currently most research is centered around increasing the use of serotonin, an amine that stimulates nerves. Many neuropsychiatrists and researchers believe that underutilized serotonin is responsible for depression, irritability, and even some forms of anxiety. This is certainly the thrust of the new psychiatric medications introduced in the last seven years. At the time of this writing, these "Specific Serotonin Reuptake Inhibitors" include Prozac, Zoloft, Paxil, and Effexor—all brand names. Many individuals have been helped by these new medications.

Despite the value of medication for depression, as well as the group of Benzodiazeapines specifically designed to combat anxiety, a few patients may experience some degree of sedation and/or a tendency to addiction, fueling the nature-nurture controversy as to whether we are more than the sum of our chemistry.

A second part of this controversy, often underplayed, is the question, How much does our life experience, especially during our developmental years through puberty, affect and change our very brain chemistry, which has been thought of as purely hereditary? In addition, can trauma experienced during any part of life do the same? These questions require further research, so the "nature-nurture" controversy will continue until we settle on the idea that *both* play a part in the development of our personalities and character.

Anorexia nervosa, for the most part (90 percent) develops between the ages of eleven and twenty-two. Puberty through adolescence are the ages in which most hormonal changes take place, affecting moods and behaviors. Just walk into a junior high school and watch the restlessness, giggling, and general diffused energy, both verbal and physical, emanating from the children. Girls experience difficulties during puberty not only from the physical aspect, but from mood changes as well. It is easy to "blame" these mood changes on the biological-endocrine-hormonal changes. From a biological point of view, most of the changes that are in play during this time may cause or aggravate any tendency toward emotional destabilization.

The earliest years of life may be a better time to evaluate purely hereditary tendencies toward mood and anxiety disorders. When we see the onset of the illness at fifteen years of age or older, we know that there is an interplay between hereditary tendency and the adolescent's family experience.

Advances in genetic counseling enable us to understand that genetic diseases ranging from diabetes to polycystic kidney disease are passed on through the gene pool at different rates of risk, depending on the disease and the family members who have suffered from it. When a couple decides to have a child, they may have some sense of the risk involved that one of their children may contract a genetic disease. This rarely influences the decision whether to have a child or not, it just alerts the future parents to the possibility that the child may develop the disease in question.

We rarely question the psychological/psychiatric disorders unless one occurs. Then the family consults a psychiatrist, who asks, "Are there members of your family who are alcoholic, depressed, suicidal, anxious, phobic?" It is at this point that the possibility of inherited psychiatric disorder chemistry begins to be estimated. Alas, "estimated" is still all we are capable of doing. The implication of a probable inherited condition is likely to imply the prompt use of medication as well as psychotherapy to treat the disorder. Patients and their family may have moral and religious conflicts about the use of a medication that affects mood, anxiety, or personality changes.

A major issue that continually confronts those of us involved in the diagnosis and treatment of mental disorders is: If the disorders are hereditary/organic in nature at the time they are diagnosed, is their organicity specific to this particular disorder—anorexia, obsessive-compulsive, phobia, etc.—or is it an organic subdivision of a larger disorder, the two largest being "Depressive" and "Anxiety" disorders? The diagnosis falls into two categories, the first being the specific symptom (Axis 1), "Anorexia nervosa," and the second, more general umbrella category (Axis II), "Depressive disorder" or "Anxiety disorder." This second category is often more related to biochemical heredity, although this conclusion is still in dispute among researchers.

The implications of someone having a biochemical disorder would seem to suggest treating it solely with medication. Many years ago, I found myself lecturing with a psychopharmacologist who stated some outcomes of such medication treatment that puzzled him. He was treating patients who had bulimia nervosa with medication (mono amine oxidase inhibitors). These patients stopped their bingeing and vomiting within two to three weeks of taking their medications. After six weeks of being symptom-free, they stopped taking their medication and resumed the bingeing and vomiting. However, after relapsing, they did not resume their medications. Why not? The physician's assumption was that they had sought his help to get rid of their symptoms. He never stated to them that the medication was a "cure" but that while taking it they might become symptom-free. The patients did not complain about unwanted side effects that could make the medication more trouble than help.

What the physician did not take into consideration was that to these patients their disease had become part of their life, their identity, and assisted them in creating a sense of emotional balance.

Rationally, they wanted to get rid of the disease; but emotionally, they missed it, as if they had lost a close friend. Many patients in treatment talk about "missing their illness" or being afraid to let go of it. The medication treated the "drive" to pursue the symptomatic behavior, but not the psychological attachment people develop toward their own familiar behaviors, healthy or not. This is the task of the psychotherapist and the environment—family, friends, work setting, and so on. The victim must undergo a "transfer of attachment" from the unhealthy behavior to persons in her life. Even if the patient had a purely hereditary predisposition to her disorder, once she developed the disordered behavior and became used to it and the reactions of those around her, then the psychological attachment had to be addressed by a trusted person or persons.

The physical symptoms which develop during the course of anorexia hamper the patient's "availability" to receive treatment.

They also frighten and anger those who would treat them, as well as their family, friends, and community. The apparent physical damage of starvation/emaciation, and the knowledge that medical damage is ongoing during the illness, creates yet another chasm between the anorexic and those involved with her.

The Biological Development of Anorexia Nervosa

Lowering one's weight is serious medicine. Dropping weight too rapidly, or reducing one's weight below what the body demands as minimal weight, triggers many biological changes. The most common changes found among girls and women with anorexia nervosa include:

- Bradycardia, a slowing of the heart rate from an average of 72 bpm to 38 bpm and even lower, causing the risk of dangerous arrhythmia, or lethal insufficiency.
- Cardiac atrophy, or shrinking of the size of the heart.
- Severe hypotension, blood pressure low enough to put someone in a state of shock.
- Hypothermia, a drop in body temperature to 95° Fahrenheit or even lower, causing temporary or permanent loss of peripheral vascular circulation, which in turn causes numbness and frostbite in the hands and feet.
- Dehydration of the cerebral cortex, or shrinking in the size of the brain. This may account for the personality changes we see in all starving persons, including those who are forced into famine and starvation.

The most commonly known biological change that takes place in the female body during starvation is the shutdown of the reproductive system. This includes the lowering of estrogen production, which gives the body many instructions, cessation of the menstrual cycle, reduced breast size, diminished vaginal secretions, disruption of ovulation and menstruation, and the absence of all desire for sexual activity.

While these are the most well publicized physical effects, when starvation and emaciation occur over a short period of time, reproductive dysfunctions usually return to normal once a healthy weight has been stabilized. Very few anorexics have ever been frightened enough by the *biological* dangers to abandon their symptomatic behavior.

All the above symptoms are starvation symptoms, not limited to those who starve from anorexia. Most of these symptoms add to fatigue, insomnia, irritability, rigidity, and general mood changes. The individual who already suffers from any of these will find that preexisting personality characteristics have been intensified, as has the person's general pattern of emotional separation from others. Others around her who witness the visual self-destruction going on, as well as becoming aware of the deterioration of her health, are separated from her by their fear, their rage, and their frustration.

The self-destructive behavior of the anorexic affects family and professionals in psychology, nutrition, and medicine alike. Professionals have a difficult time deciding whether it is the patient or the disease they are fighting. Although this disease usually has some hereditary or biological roots, the disease itself complicates any biological roots by adding its own biological changes, as well as deepening any psychological problems that would make one predisposed to it. It would not be fair to end this chapter without adding that the "culture of feminine thinness" acts as a "hereditary" root. All females born into the culture of feminine thinness are rendered more prone to develop it.

The net result of all these factors is a person with an illness that creates more divisiveness among those who are involved with her than any other illness that comes to mind.

LOUISE

Girls brought up in this culture—including those with hereditary predispositions, anxiety disorders, depressive disorders, or a combination—do not necessarily develop anorexia nervosa, other related eating disorders, or other psychologically based behavior disorders. There are ways in which we can identify predisposed children and modify parenting to minimize the change that they will succumb to these anxiety-depressive disorders.

Let's take the case of Louise. She was a colicky baby, had night terrors as a child, had a difficult time staying in her own bed in her own room at night, was afraid to be left with baby-sitters, and vomited out of anxiety the first day of kindergarten.

Louise's parents consulted me during her first week of kindergarten and provided a clear history of an anxious child, probably anxious from birth.

Louise's mother described herself as an anxious person, "a worrier," as she put it. Louise's father described himself as an independent, risk-taking man, a lawyer who took on controversial cases and thrived on the challenges his work provided. He was one of nine children; both his parents had to work, so there was no time for worry or indecision.

A further history of his extended family revealed two brothers suffering from alcoholism, a third brother who committed suicide, a sister with postpartum depression with her second child, two sisters who were divorced—one coping well, one poorly; and two brothers he regarded as happily married and with successful careers. His parents were hardworking people who ran a dry cleaning store together, where many of the children spent after-school time doing homework, or helping out. He said that his parents were working-class heroes and that their only complaint was fatigue.

Louise's mother described her own family as much smaller. She had one older brother. Louise's father was a mechanical engineer who worked hard but reiterated his worries about getting laid off or fired for as long as she could remember. Her mother was at home; her brother, who was "odd and introverted," left college and had taken many jobs, which never lasted long (less than a year). He was living with his parents at the age of thirty-nine.

At this point it becomes obvious that for one reason or another there are many people in Louise's gene pool with a variety of problems often caused by depression and anxiety. Louise's own history suggests that she has been an anxious child as far back as she and her parents can remember.

Will Louise develop anorexia nervosa sometime between puberty and late adolescence? It is probable that our culture will channel her anxiety and possibly her depression (children who know that they are less happy and calm than other children become depressed and feel inferior about the contrast) into a behavioral-emotional disorder. Anorexia is the most likely candidate, but bulimia, obesity, obsessive-compulsive disorder, phobia, or severe feelings of inferiority, depression, alienation, and other problems may result if they are not dealt with as early as possible.

Heading   Off   Biological   Predispositions   Toward Psychological Disorders

Before a full-blown psychological disorder develops in reaction to a child's "not feeling right," several preventative steps can be taken.

1. Acknowledge the child's "not feeling well," whether this is identifiable as fearfulness, insomnia, timidity, shyness, panic attacks, overdependency on being with a parent, etc. Acknowledge it to yourself as a parent so that you won't take it as acting out on the part of the child, or an insult to you. Describe it to the child, and ask the child what it feels like to be having those feelings. Let the child talk, and nod your head in agreement that "that must feel awful." This creates a bond

between parent and child where disordered behavior usually separates them. This bond prevents the child's pain from "going underground" into the subconscious and becoming "strange" or developing disordered behavior.

2. Confer with your spouse, parents, friends, clergyperson, or all of the above, so that you will be supported, and won't feel isolated and frightened by your child's behavior.

3. Read all you can on the subject of eating disorders and use your common sense when interpreting what you read and what you hear from professionals.

The "nature-nurture" controversy, or heredity versus family, environment, and life experience as the prime influence on personality development and emotional stability, will and should continue until we have many more answers. Then we will have to ask how much nature can affect nurture, and visa versa. For example, someone with a genetic propensity toward anxiety could be perceived as irritating to the family, who might then retaliate with hostility. This, in turn, further intensifies the child's anxiety. Conversely, anxious parents can create insecurity in an otherwise relaxed child. The fact that one's biological parents usually create the child's environment as well as his or her genetic makeup makes it hard to delineate where nature ends and nurture begins.

9

WHEN CAUSES COLLIDE

A *Chain of Experiences*

WHAT causes anorexia nervosa?" I have been asked this question by members of the media and guests at parties. Every host would like to hear one answer, one cause, and hopefully, one cure. "Why do one, or even two children in the same family develop it, while others don't?"

In this chapter, I hope to clarify the chain of experiences necessary to develop this illness. Often the chain has different links but leads to the same place.

Anxiety is an uncomfortable state. My thesaurus offers the following synonyms for the word: "Anguish, apprehension, concern, dread, fear, foreboding, misgiving, trepidation, wariness, and worry." I am sure that more unpleasant words can be added to this list.

When we experience anxiety, we need to assign a reason. If we establish the cause for its existence, we can develop a strategy to "make it go away." The reason does not have to be accurate or correct. If we believe the reason is real, we can then attempt to plan our strategy, and when accomplished, we expect the anxiety to go away. If we cannot discover, "invent," or rationalize a reason for this anxiety, we find it unbearable. Therefore, we always succeed at finding a reason, no matter how unusual our assigned cause may be.

Individuals may often employ the same reasons and strategy that cause the feelings of anxiety in order to make the feelings go away. In anorexia, a girl may get upset about the way a dress fits her, a comment someone made about her having gained weight, or being jealous about a friend's appearance. This experience may have caused her to worry that she would become increasingly unattractive to boys and that girls may abandon her for more "popular-looking" friends. As her anxiety attacks become more frequent, for a variety of adolescent causes, she mentally puts them into the "I'm too fat" track, which implies that if only she were thin, her anxiety would go away.

After a period of weeks, she isn't even identifying her feeling as anxiety. Instead, she has "abbreviated" it to "I feel fat" or "I'm having a fat day." It is at this point that she starts to anticipate "feeling fat" and is continuously dieting, exercising, and taking other steps to control her weight *before* she can feel (anxious) fat.

Fat has now become an *obsession*. After all, anything or anyone (including herself) may bring on the feeling again. She has invented the cause for all her anxiety, present and future, and must take increasing steps to ward off this intrusive feeling.

The obvious implications of this process are that she will desperately pursue weight-losing behavior without regard to her appearance, her health, or the opinion of others.

If her feelings of femininity are substantial, her changing appearance in the mirror might act as a brake on the weight plunge. If her feelings of femininity are not substantial, she will disregard her increasingly diminishing physical femininity and perceive her shrinking breasts as "getting rid of fat," her loss of her menstrual period as proof that she is succeeding in becoming thin enough, her emaciated torso and limbs as providing an ever-increasing buffer between her current appearance and the danger of becoming fat. Trying to look more feminine might have been the reason at the beginning for losing weight, but the original reason and her thoughts of femininity have become obscured by the obsessional state of mind she now finds herself in.

This shift involves a severe change in focus from "outward" to "inward." The extreme form of turning inward is a *narcissistic state,* which puts a barrier between oneself and others. The narcissist no longer cares about others, except for their positive and negative reactions and the consequences they will have on the narcissist, which is the only way that the obsessed "care" about others.

Anorexia nervosa either creates a narcissistic state of mind or intensifies one that already exists. A major part of treatment, which will be discussed in later chapters, deals with reducing the "narcissistic/obsessional" state—the extreme "turning inward" and away from attachments to others.

This change usually begins during stage three of the illness—the Assertive Stage (see chapter 3). One way to determine how much narcissistic/obsessiveness has developed is to evaluate the intensity of the defiance and secretiveness a subject uses to defend her illness.

ELLEN

Ellen was brought to treatment at the age of fourteen. She was five foot seven and weighed seventy-six pounds. She was cheerful, outgoing, and claimed that she never weighed herself and didn't care about her weight. Even at this point one could see that Ellen had been pretty at her original weight of one hundred and ten pounds. Her mother showed me earlier photos to convey her heartbreak at Ellen's deteriorating appearance.

Ellen had begun to lose weight a year earlier. Her parents barely noticed the loss of the first ten pounds. She had always been a competent child, always gave the correct, appropriate response in any given situation. It was difficult for them even to notice her weight loss at first since they were not used to being vigilant about how she took care of herself. It was when she had lost twenty pounds and weighed only ninety pounds that the school nurse sent a letter home calling Ellen's weight loss into question and recommending that she be seen by a physician.

Ellen had initially experienced admiration from her peer group. She had the willpower to resist eating rich foods and could casually lose weight without even talking about it. After all, our culture dictates that all women should be as thin as possible, and though we see, read about, and hear lots of talk about being "toned," the not-so-hidden implication is never missed by young girls or women.

As Ellen continued her drop in both weight and size, her friends' approval turned to worry, criticism, and finally to anger at what was in their eyes unreasonable, foolish, stubborn behavior on her part. Ellen "defied" their comments by ignoring their advice and scolding.

Secretly, perhaps unconsciously, Ellen was enjoying her newfound independence. Usually, she complied with the wishes of others. Now she remained morally comfortable in the knowledge that she was following the cultural directive to be devoid of fat. She inwardly guarded her caloric intake while outwardly acting (in statements and attitude) as if it didn't matter. Her obsession with losing weight was her biggest secret. Her assertiveness in defense of her illness was charming and undetectable. She blithely told others, including her parents, that "there's nothing to worry about. I eat healthy foods and my appearance and weight are fine."

The "Assertive Stage" is usually quite a battle between the anorexic and those around her, but in Ellen's case it was more of a battle with her own guardedness. When Ellen was in treatment, she was extremely guarded about voicing her thoughts and feelings. It was quite a task for her to open up and talk about her anorexia. Because she did let down her guard, her weight climbed from seventy-seven to one hundred pounds before she temporarily (for one year) refused to gain any more weight. As Ellen finally let go of her need to "turn inward," she gained weight and her mental health improved. Normally, treatments produce weight gain without a concomitant improvement in mental health. In Ellen's case, she was bargaining with her weight. She would gain weight and keep it on in exchange for feeling better. (Treatments that merely coerce weight without an improvement in mental health are discussed in chapter 11.)

Incest Trauma

Often when we report that a person has "incest" in his or her background, we tend to perceive it as another stressful experience, but we may inadvertently trivialize it as just one more unfortunate event or series of events in the patient's life. I use the phrase "incest trauma" so that we don't lose track of the nature of this particularly horrifying and destructive experience, whether it is one episode (rarely) or a series of episodes that goes on for years.

Many people have asked me if there is a connection between incest trauma and anorexia nervosa and I am left with the equivocating answer, "Sometimes." I would like to clarify here what that "Sometimes" means in the causal relationship between incest trauma and the onset of anorexia nervosa.

When a parent fondles or "invades" the body of a son or daughter, the child immediately understands that *there is no one out there to protect me*. This inference, of course, includes all members of the family. If the incestuous assault is between father and daughter, the daughter has nowhere to turn. Her first response is to blame herself. Children are always more comfortable blaming themselves when harmed by their parents, for two reasons: if it's the child's fault, then the child can behave differently to stop the parent's assaultive behavior; if it's the child's fault, then the child still can view her parent as competent. Not having a competent parent is close to unthinkable for a child, for it leaves her feeling parentless.

Her second response might be to ask her mother to "save her" from her father's behavior, but even the youngest girl who can verbally explain this to her mother fears her mother will blame her, call her a liar, or accuse her of competing for her father's attention. So the child has nowhere to go. She must turn inward to contrive an acceptable meaning for the act, or else forget it ever happened — even if the trauma is repeated, it can be repeatedly forgotten.

What is not forgotten is the child's feeling that there is no one to turn to "out there." A premature independence must be developed. And she can only accept support, comfort, and reassurance from herself, since no one else is trustworthy. Her methods of self-soothing may involve seeking to be the best at something: schoolwork, athletics, and of course, thinness. She may also turn to obsessive-compulsive rituals to make all her imaginary successes feel real.

JESSICA

Jessica was five years old when her father first raped her. He continued until she was twelve years old and she got her first menstrual period.

By day, he was an attentive, if not a warm father. He taught her how to fish, how to sail, even how to use a bow and arrow. He taught her how to ride a bike, to observe and identify birds. At night, he would enter her room, and when he was finished, leave without a word. She thought that these strange and painful experiences were something that she was supposed to adjust to, even though she continued to dread them. She thought about telling her mother, but perhaps her mother knew about them already, would think her a complainer, and be annoyed with her. On other occasions when she wanted to bring up the subject, it occurred to her that her mother might be mad at her for having a "special" relationship with her father, or think that she was lying about the whole thing.

Jessica began to invest rituals that she hoped would spare her her father's attentions. He didn't show up every night, but rather several times a week, and she developed a host of personal superstitions to ward off his appearance on any one night. These superstitions might involve the color of the clothing she would wear on a particular day of the week, the route she would take to school, special ribbons she would put in her hair, and others too numerous to mention. When her father failed to show up during a particular night, she would review the superstitions she had contrived that day and try them again the next day. If they failed to ward off the event, she would double up on some of them while eliminating others. She was very involved in finding a "magic" solution to her problem, which she believed no person could help her solve.

Jessica's skepticism about people helping her with problems spread to all areas of personal assistance just as her superstitiousness spread to all sorts of behaviors. Indeed, she was quite detached from others except in the most superficial and conversational ways. But she appeared outgoing and friendly to children her own age, teachers, and even her family. No one knew how much of her thoughts and activities involved protecting herself through magic or superstition, even though the results of her efforts afforded no protection.

When Jessica turned twelve and her father stopped his nighttime behavior, she was sure it was due to some successful combination of superstitious rituals. His behavior had been going on for seven years. Just as her behaviors had not worked before age twelve, everything she did worked afterward. He never came to her bedroom again. But her whole orientation toward her own security was based on the magic she had developed over the years. Now Jessica was almost consciously looking for a new danger to justify her continued use of magic.

By the time she had turned thirteen, all her friends were talking about the dangers of becoming overweight, getting thick thighs, big tummies, and so on. The "magic" she was hearing about involved restrictive eating and exercise. Jessica liked this idea. It was more certain than her seven years of invented superstition had been. She was a slender thirteen-year-old; five foot four, one hundred pounds, long flowing red hair with subtle freckles to match.

Soon Jessica began to restrict her calories and had more success with her weight loss than she ever had with keeping her father out of her bedroom. This new behavior felt very powerful to her. She continued losing weight and was admonished by her mother after the first ten pounds disappeared. She was warned by her doctor shortly thereafter. Her friends made disparaging comments about this eighty-pound girl. She was thrilled but showed none of her happiness to anyone. When the boys in her school made it clear that they thought that she was ugly, she was ecstatic: "No boys, no men, no fathers, no more rape!"

Being raped by her father had been the most frightening and painful experience of Jessica's life. Like all incest victims, she partially blamed herself. She wondered, "Perhaps I behaved in the wrong way. Perhaps this happens to every daughter and it doesn't bother them. They just don't talk about it. Maybe it's me. I can't cope."

Nevertheless, it remained the most intense experience of her life. She recalled with horror that sometimes when she was being raped, she experienced a "buzzy, tingly" feeling that felt good. This made her, in her own mind, a co-conspirator in the whole experience — more proof she was the one to be blamed.

But when the raping stopped, Jessica was faced with the problem of replacing this feeling of intensity and danger that had dominated her thoughts for years. She would need another focus, another obsession — another danger.

Becoming thin would do fine. She would substitute "remaining the same weight, or gaining weight," for rape. She would substitute "losing weight" for having her father not come into her bedroom. She would invent new rituals related to weight loss such as restricting her eating, exercising, taking diet pills, laxatives, even reducing the amount of liquids she was drinking, in the mistaken hope that it would reduce her weight further.

In effect, Jessica, because of her history of being an incest victim which turned her inward from those around her, was ready to transfer her mental energy from protecting herself from being raped by her father to becoming too fat, a threat the "culture of thinness" for women had taught her.

With the speed that an upper-class college student uses to transfer credits for advanced standing, Jessica moved quickly through the four stages of anorexia and became immediately a severe, rapid-weight-losing, detached, defiant anorexic, at the fourth stage.

It would take years of therapy to help Jessica disclose, understand, develop a trusting therapeutic relationship; to use healthy dependence and attachment to replace her inward-turning attempts at safety with interpersonal safety, which would allow her to relinquish her anorexia nervosa and not replace it with other obsessional targets to regulate her anxiety.

10

ANOREXIA

AND

COLLEGE ATTENDANCE

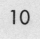NE of the greatest changes an adolescent experiences is leaving home to attend a residential college. Unless she has attended boarding school, this is her first time away from home living with her parents, a change that implies that "Things will never be the same again." Separation from parents infers growth and maturity. If the adolescent went to summer camp, that experience might have provoked anxiety. Leaving for college implies "moving out."

When an adolescent feels secure in her relationship with her parents, she feels safer leaving for college, knowing that security is only a phone call away. When an adolescent does not feel secure with her parents, or not at peace with them, she feels that her childhood or her adolescence has "incomplete" aspects. She is not ready for independence yet, she wants to cling to her home and family. At college away from home, this girl is at risk for developing anorexia, bulimia, and other emotional problems. Researchers have suggested as many as 19 percent of college coeds have one form of eating disorder or another.

Should My Child Go Away to College?

First, we might look at the question, Who should go away to a residential college, and who shouldn't? This question is important with girls who have a history of eating disorders, although other emotional problems may apply as well. We all start with the assumption that if a family can afford it, and their daughter or son is academically qualified for college, she or he will enroll. As a culture, we also assume that a residential college, away from home, is preferable. Yet even if academic abilities and family finances make it possible, many adolescents are too emotionally immature to make the requisite break with home.

The adolescent's security for herself and her family is one criterion. There are others. How ready is she for the absence of daily support, affection, and the end of supervision? College freshmen are not grown-ups. Regardless of whether it is politically correct to call them "college women" or "college men," at eighteen or nineteen they are still adolescents—part child, part adult—continuing their struggle between the two polarities. "Politically correct" designations may create further demands on them and confer an unreal status that supports them artificially.

Notable among freshmen in particular, and older students as well, are the excesses to which some students will go to prove that they can do what "Mommy and Daddy" never let them do. Some of the behaviors that reflect these fears are drinking to excess, vomiting, drugging to amnesia, paralysis, temporary blindness, and other general nonfunctional states. Fear of losing their parents' protection, fear of not knowing how they will fare after college, fear of how they will fit into the world of work and careers, fear of intimacy with the opposite sex, need for healthy friendships with the same sex—all of these demands require developing maturity and an adult identity, which entails adult responsibilities . . . and they've just left home! They know that the clock is ticking, set for four years from their admission to college. If the protective "bubble" of college is scary, what happens when the "maturity clock" runs out, they graduate, and the bubble bursts?

Obviously, we can't establish criteria that might well eliminate 30 percent of college-bound high school students from applying to residential colleges. Yet we must attempt to evaluate students so that we do not send high school graduates off to likely failure. Colleges take great pains to establish the suitability of students for admission to their institutions; they use grade-point averages, class ranking, SAT scores, extracurricular activities, and recommendations. Colleges ask students to write essays about themselves, and they usually conduct personal interviews with candidates.

Parents then must establish their own requirements to determine whether their child will have more emotional success at a residential college as opposed to a commuter or community college. The first assumption we should consider dropping is, "Everyone who can afford it goes away to a residential college."

It should not be considered less desirable for a student to commute to college or to go to a college near enough to home (two hours by car, bus, or train) so that they can return on weekends when they want to or need to.

If a student has suffered from an eating disorder during her high school years and has not yet recovered by the beginning of her senior year in high school, she becomes a high risk for relapse during her freshman year at college. This situation is so prevalent that it requires careful scrutiny on the part of the girl's family.

Another warning sign may be what is commonly referred to as "senioritis," when a student's work drops off sharply during her senior year, especially if it happens before acceptance to college. If her behavior reaches the level that her graduation is in jeopardy, she may be indicating more than just indifference to schoolwork because she has "escaped" from her high school's control and will be leaving for college.

It is difficult for parents to distinguish between adolescent rebellious exuberance and signs of impending trouble. Each parent must view the senior's behavior in the context of her past emotional history and the health of the family system.

JOY

Joy had been diagnosed as having anorexia nervosa during her junior year in high school. She had been hospitalized three times for malnutrition and dehydration. In addition to restricting her eating, she abused laxatives and exercised to exhaustion. Two of her three hospitalizations were emergency admissions after she collapsed. When the hospital staff realized that Joy was a danger to herself and had provoked her own crisis, they transferred her to the psychiatric unit, where she remained for a period of three to four weeks in order to stabilize her eating, treat her laxative addiction, and monitor her fluid intake to avoid dehydration.

After she was discharged from the third hospital admission, she remained in treatment with an outpatient psychotherapist and her parents believed that the worst was over, since this time she hadn't lost any weight. Once at home, however, her laxative abuse continued (secretly) as did her exercising. The plans were for Joy to go away to a prestigious college; even though she was still symptomatic during her senior year of high school, when she was accepted to this college, the whole family rejoiced. But, the college was some eight hundred miles from home. This would make casual trips back too time-consuming and expensive. Joy was advised by her therapist that she was not ready to leave home, since he knew that she was still symptomatic. He demanded that she tell her parents in a family therapy session about the status of her eating disorder.

They met the following week and Joy admitted to the continued use of laxatives, and exhaustive exercising when no one else was home. Her parents were shocked and disappointed. They yelled at her and demanded, "How could you be so stupid?" After they calmed down, they decided that since her weight had remained normal, she would move on with the other successful students in her graduating class and go the college.

During her first month at college, two of Joy's dorm mates called her parents to say they were worried about her.

Her new college friends never saw her eat—in the dining room or anywhere else. They also noticed that she was becoming thinner and looked malnourished. They didn't want to report her to Student Services until they called her home first.

Joy's mother thanked the girls for their concern and hung up. During dinner that evening, she broached the subject to her husband. "Two of Joy's roommates phoned today." He stopped eating and stared at her, waiting for the next sentence. "They were worried that she was starving herself." He dropped his fork. It clattered loudly as it hit the plate. He looked down, sighing in anger and frustration. "I guess we shouldn't have let her go." His wife sat watching her husband go through changes in attitude toward his daughter. He put his hands on his temples. "How could she be so stupid? How could she do this to herself . . . and us?"

After relating this conversation during a therapy session, Joy's mother asked the therapist what they should do.

In reviewing Joy's history with both parents, the therapist concluded that Joy had been "stubborn," whether in a concession to her father's anger or because she still felt trapped in her disease though she had gained her weight back. Her outward appearance had been deceptive, allaying the fears of her parents. Inwardly, she was still sick, unable to cope with her fears, and abbreviating all of her fears into that one catch-all, "feeling fat."

"Joy is a chronic anorexic," the therapist commented. "That means she would resist all efforts to change her eating behavior and weight with all her resourcefulness and energy."

"You make it sound hopeless," her mother commented.

"I don't know if it's hopeless. What I do know is that it will take an enormous amount of energy to change the triangle."

Her father looked up at him with raised eyebrows. "What do you mean by 'change the triangle'?"

"Right now, your daughter feels like she is part of an isosceles triangle. You remember, that's the triangle that has two long legs and one short one connecting them, like one face of an Egyptian pyramid, if we made it twice as tall, but no wider at the base."

"What does geometry have to do with my daughter's weight loss?" Her father was annoyed.

"Your daughter feels like it's her and her anorexia against the world."

"It sounds like she is more attached to it than us, or even the rest of her activities."

"She is."

"How do we make her more attached to us than it?"

"It's an ambitious goal. We compete with it. We let her know what this best friend of hers is, what 'it' says to her."

"Can we do this at college or does she have to come home?"

"Frankly," the therapist began, "I wish that you and she had chosen a college nearer to your home. If she is to stay at college—and ideally it's a good starting place—you will have to do a lot of commuting. You will have to risk her displeasure, anger, and occasionally her rage at your intruding into her college life. You will have to continually remind her that if this intruding fails, she will have to come home, and if that fails, she will have to go to a hospital."

They both looked exhausted as they listened to a plan that made sense to them but required that they change their relationship with their daughter and spend so much time and energy fighting a problem they thought professionals would repair for them.

Joy's father asked, "How do we 'intrude,' as you put it, without her hating us? If she is more attached to her patterns than she is to us," he was becoming tearful, "then how do we win her over with anything that sounds as unattractive as this posture you're advocating?"

"We are not talking about being nasty, or harsh, or mean. We are talking about setting firm, explainable, reasonable limits and demands. We are also talking about caring, protecting, loving, and communicating intensely with someone who has isolated herself from close communication with others."

"But isn't this an age where young people are striving for more independence? Isn't this a backward move in her development?" her mother inquired.

"Your daughter, like all late adolescents, can only achieve a truly healthy independence if she has already achieved an adequate period where she has been healthily dependent. Most anorexics miss that period, so, yes, we are going backwards, or regressing, treating her as if she were younger. This helps to build in that missing piece of dependence that causes her to depend on her anorexia instead of both of you. She has obviously warded off any attempts by both of you—and me—to lure her away from her sick dependency to a healthier one. We now have to increase our effort, include the college counseling staff in what we are doing, and enlist their efforts to support our strategy. This will create a consistency all around Joy that will become irresistible and finally more attractive than her anorexia."

"Are we talking about a disease or a lollipop?" Joy's father interjected. "You talk about competing with her anorexia. Aren't we, her parents, more attractive to her than a set of rules that she has made up?"

"I'm afraid that the answer is no, since she listens to that anorexic voice more than anyone she knows. We mustn't confuse attraction with love. Despite her love for you, she became compelled, lured, conditioned—drawn into the mental system of these ideas that have more control over her than you and your wife have. Your task, and the task of all those involved in helping Joy, is to offer her more emotional security than this disease does. We must win what is, as you put it, a competition."

Joy's father just shook his head as he stared at the floor.

The next day, Joy had a telephone conversation with her mother. She was told that her parents would notify the school about her condition and would request that Student Health Services be responsible for weighing her weekly and reporting that weight to a counselor, who would work with her on a twice-a-week basis. If her weight dropped more than three pounds, she would be taken out of school and brought home. The counseling department suggested that Joy join the Eating Disorders Group at the student center, as well. In addition, Joy would be followed up by the college physician, who would monitor her general health and review it with Joy. Her parents decided to visit her twice a month on the weekends. If they could get there on a Friday, they would have sessions with Joy and her counselor.

The Role of the College

Colleges vary in their ability and resources to assist students with psychological problems. Some have a large enough counseling staff to see any student in need of help on a regular weekly basis; some can only make referrals to outside, local therapists, and even for this service, students may have to wait a long time for an appointment. This becomes another criterion for parents when selecting a residential college for their daughter who may have recurrent emotional problems.

A proportion of the female students in all colleges suffer from eating disorders (anorexia and bulimia). As a result, college staffs once oblivious to the problem are paying some attention to it now, in addition to the attention they pay to general psychological problems that students bring with them when they enter college, or develop during the time they are there. We used to talk about special interest groups at colleges as clubs. Although these still exist in many colleges, special interest groups are more likely to be "special problem-centered groups" than before. And again, staffs have different degrees of specialization in eating disorders. Colleges also vary in how pro-active and regulatory they are about allowing students with emotional problems, especially eating disorders, to remain on campus. Some colleges suspend or expel students with eating disorders if they seem to be in jeopardy; others ignore the issue.

Today's college cafeteria can be far from relaxing for college women. The boys/men haven't changed much from high school. They eat to satisfy their hunger. Adequacy or competitiveness simply does not enter their minds.

College girls/women have an entirely different experience in the cafeteria. It is a testing ground for willpower. Girls notice what other girls have on their trays, how much they eat, and when they're eating. There is eating talk. "I really ate too much this weekend at the frat party. It will take me two weeks to make up for it." Comments that are self-deprecatory are common. "I wish I had your figure."

The recovering anorexic is particularly vulnerable to all of this talk. It makes her feel that she should "get back in the game." She may feel resentful. Many anorexics have asked me, "Why do I have to gain weight while everyone around me has the right to lose weight?"

This is where parents become confused. We all naturally assume that when someone is "recovering," they are improving and are pleased that they are "better" than they used to be. They suffer less, are overcoming a handicap, and would never want to return to their "sicker" state. To understand the concept of "jealousy" of those sicker than ourselves, we have to apply an addiction model. The most common addiction is smoking. No one is more upset than the recent quitter when others are smoking around him. He makes speeches about how he quit and berates those who haven't managed to do so. A substantial part of his righteous energy comes from his jealousy that he cannot smoke. He may have demanded this of himself but he's stuck with it. He did it because he believed it was healthy for him to stop smoking—but he still wants to.

An anorexic in the early stages of gaining weight, and even the early stages of attaining her goal weight, still feels shaky about the loss of her security system and jealous of other anorexics or girls who might look anorexic to her.

If the social norm for college women is to stay as thin as possible, as it is for the rest of girls and women in society, then the anorexic is jealous that she is left out of a competition she used to be the best in. It takes awhile for her to replace the anorexia with more realistic ways of attaining balance, security, and a sense of adequacy. College-age students are more intense about their feelings than they will be as they mature beyond the college years. This intensity, peer pressure, and the recovering anorexic's own intensity make the residential college environment a more difficult place to heal when the wound is still tender and subject to abuse.

The abuse I am referring to here is the "public eating" of low-calorie foods done by women in many college cafeterias, the diet talk, and the self-criticism others make of their "overweight."

Residential colleges, while allowing freedoms many students don't have at home, encourage growth and maturity in most who attend. Sadly, those who fall into excessively destructive behaviors were not mature enough, or healthy enough, to leave home in the first place.

11

TREATMENT CHOICES

WHEN someone is diagnosed as having cancer, they may become terrified, depressed, numb, or go into complete denial and talk as if it were a minor incident.

When persons are diagnosed with a psychiatric disorder, on the other hand, usually they are relieved that their mysterious feelings and thoughts can be demystified and hopefully diminish and eventually go away.

But when girls and young women are diagnosed as having anorexia nervosa, most go into a conscious denial concerning the diagnosis, not to themselves but to others. They often feel caught, discovered, cornered, or trapped. These individuals, unlike those mentioned above, are not ready to become patients, not ready for treatment, and will not benefit from treatment *until* they are ready.

Medically speaking, we cannot wait them out until they are ready for treatment, because the clock is ticking and the scale indicator is dropping. They will run out of pounds—and the ability to survive.

So, treatment will have to begin before they are ready, before they wish it to begin. We cannot leave them in charge of deciding when it should begin.

There are a variety of ways of treating anorexia nervosa, some distinct, some a blend of several approaches. Some allow for more patient autonomy, some allow for none. All of these treatments have their place in the spectrum. The task of the evaluator is to select the appropriate treatment for the patient at the time she is seen. At some point, progress—or the lack of it—may indicate that another form of treatment be attempted. Indeed, selecting a form of treatment and deciding when to change is a process of educated trial and error.

For the bewildered family and victim, it is helpful to classify this treatment into several distinct categories. The types listed below do not include all those available and the reader is invited to explore further, using other sources.

Individual Psychotherapy

Individual psychotherapy can take various forms. It is recommended for the most motivated, the most ready for treatment, and usually for the anorexic who is least endangered by low weight and its health-related problems, has an early diagnosis, and has the smallest number of "treatment failures" in the past.

We will turn to this again in the discussion of specific patients later in the chapters.

Group Psychotherapy

This is usually an adjunct to individual psychotherapy, both in inpatient settings, such as psychiatric hospitals, and in outpatient settings at treatment centers. It is an extremely useful method, since it helps many anorexics who feel misunderstood and alone with their problems share with others who have similar experiences. It can be powerful as a therapeutic tool—even for the long-term patient—since it involves peer support, peer confrontation, and little room for "fooling oneself." The risk with group therapy is that those who have less experience with the disease, and those who are the youngest, may learn new ways to lose weight. They may become the victims of "symptom pooling." It is incumbent on the group leader to assemble a group whose members are at similar places in their illness and age to avoid this risk.

This last observation is not an indictment of group therapy. Every treatment, whether it involves medication or psychotherapy, will have some positive effects and some unwanted, undesirable side effects.

When selecting any kind of therapy for an ailment or health problem, one always weighs, on a hypothetical balance scale, the benefits versus the undesirable effects of the treatment or therapy. Cases where treatment produces no side effects are rare.

Inpatient Versus Outpatient Treatment

Today's health treatments, medical as well as psychiatric, have been strongly changed for the worse by lowered reimbursement from insurance companies who have hired health care monitoring systems to restrict payment to both physicians and patients. An enormous number of bureaucrats, at no small cost, derail monies that might be spent on health care, insist on "evaluating" the necessity of the expenditure in question, and inevitably tell both the physician and the patient that they must settle for less health care than they had before. These "hatchetmen" (and women) have become the new health care decision makers as they strip away benefits from the paying public, and deny quality treatment methods from health care providers.

The reason I take such a strong position at this point is that these changes affect all the recommendations that follow.

Two main criteria must be taken into consideration when determining whether to place a patient in a hospital program or a daycare program. The first criterion has to be: *How seriously is the patient endangered medically?*

The primary care physician must take into consideration the

height and weight of the patient, her current rate of weight loss, do a blood work-up to determine nutritional state and organ functioning, an examination to evaluate heart health, blood pressure, temperature, urine analysis, and other bodily functions—all of which the physician needs to know in order to determine the degree to which the patient is endangered.

If the patient is evaluated as being highly endangered, an acute care medical hospital might be recommended, where the patient can be most aggressively fed via intravenous or nasogastric tube. If the patient is highly resistant to treatment that would take her out of danger, then a psychiatric unit in the medical hospital would be recommended, where the staff could observe and coerce this patient in order to save her life.

If the medical danger is evaluated as being below the need for such critical intervention, but the patient's rate of weight loss is unstoppable at home and her health and weight is approaching a dangerous level, an inpatient treatment setting still might be desirable. This could be a hospital or a highly structured residential treatment center for eating disorders.

If the patient is identified early on in her weight-losing behavior, outpatient treatment—individual psychotherapy often accompanied by group therapy—would be preferable.

The second main criterion to be considered is the state of the patient's *support systems, family, and environment.* Often, the decision of how urgent, or aggressive, a treatment is necessary depends on the strength, health, and emotional resourcefulness of the family in question.

Family Therapy

A family that is beset by other health problems, medical or psychiatric, or severe marital problems, or a single-parent family without an emotional support system, will bring these problems to their role in family therapy. However, family therapy can be a powerful tool for rapid change in the relationships that foster anorexia and other emotional disorders. It is a setting where often the "unsayable" (at home) can now be said because a "referee" is present; a setting where a family can use the therapist as a teacher and role model who can step back, analyze the conflict, and resolve it.

If the family is moderately healthy, often several modes of treatment can be applied at once. Individual psychotherapy, group psychotherapy, and couples therapy for the parents.

Couples Therapy

In couples therapy, the spouses can examine their relationship with regard to mutual support, similarity of opinions about raising their child, and their ability to resolve conflicts with their child, as well as the degree of trust they both have with the care and guidance of that child. A second area to be explored is how role-appropriate each parent is with the child. Are they able to be nurturing, to set firm yet reasonable limits? Is either parent emotionally needy, and do they show their neediness to the child with the result that she becomes the nurturer? Couples therapy, as opposed to family therapy, provides privacy for parents. Children frequently know a great deal about their parents' relationships already. Separating the parents from the children for at least part of the therapy implies that there are "grown-up" issues that exclude the child. Initially, the child may resent it, but usually she is relieved to be spared unnecessary information about her parents, especially their burdens and struggles.

Another role for the couples' therapist is to evaluate the neediness that exists between the spouses. Often, the anorexic fills the parental nurturing vacuum. When the parents' therapist provides emotional support, he or she takes on the role that the anorexic child may be unwittingly playing. In this particular situation the therapist, by nurturing the parents, is releasing the child, making it possible for her to take her place in the family system.

The child (adolescent, or young adult) is now freer to develop facets of her character and personality that were forbidden by her imposed role in the family system. In individual therapy, she will be able to experiment with getting her own needs stated, expressed, and acted out as she relates to a therapist who is a nurturing personality, and who won't allow the anorexic to be the caretaker in the therapeutic relation but rather the *care receiver*, a role she is unaccustomed to. She can practice dependency with her therapist, ask advice, cry for herself, declare weakness or inability, even accept (realistic) compliments from the therapist—something she cannot do elsewhere.

Separately, her parents may be getting the same care from their therapist. In this model, the nurturing shortage available to each member of the family is being filled simultaneously by two therapists in separate settings, which facilitates rapid change in the family system.

When the anorexic is at once invited to receive from her therapist and not requested to nurture by her parents (however unconscious the request may be), she becomes able to give up her *symptomatic* (anorexic) style of getting her needs met unconsciously. At this point, the anorexic, her parents, and the family system are all in treatment and change is supported from every direction.

Self-Help Groups (without Professional Leaders)

In the 1970s, very few mental health professionals were interested in treating anorexia nervosa. I remember the tremendous number of requests for treatment I received following the publication of *The Best Little Girl in the World* (1978). I also remember calling every psychologist, psychiatrist, and social worker I knew to ask them if they would treat the overflow of potential patients who were calling me. Their answers surprised me: "No, Steve, that's not the kind of patient for me," or, "It sounds too dangerous—even hopeless," or, "I don't think these kids really want treatment. I like to treat people who want to get better; perhaps these kids belong in hospitals," or,

"I think they may all be suicidal and I'm not interested in acquiring suicidal patients."

To be fair, most of these professionals knew little or nothing about the specifics of this illness and would not feel comfortable with such patients. To add to the nonmedical therapists' worries, they didn't understand what would medically constitute endangerment and told me they might well experience fear and anger toward a patient because of his or her life-threatening symptoms.

Thus, until the beginning of the eighties there existed a disease that had no appropriate treatment setting. Outpatient psychiatrists and nonmedical therapists were untrained, and medical and psychiatric hospitals had not yet determined ways of dealing with self-starving patients who regarded the hospital staff as the enemy rather than as trying to help people.

Self-help groups sprang up in many cities, usually started by the mothers of girls with anorexia. In New Jersey, the American Anorexic Association was started by Estelle Miller; in Boston, Patricia Warner founded ANAS—Anorexia Nervosa and Associated Disorders; in Chicago, Vivian Meehan started ANAD—the National Association of Anorexia and Associated Disorders; and in Pittsburgh, Anita Sinicrope founded PENED—the Pittsburgh Educational Network for Eating Disorders.

Some of these groups formed national chapters in other cities to help beleaguered parents and relatives of anorexics. At this point, anorexics began seeking treatment for themselves, convinced by public discussions on the media that they were not "just freaks." Most notable among the national organizations formed are the National Association of Anorexia Nervosa and Associated Disorders, or ANAD, located in Highland Park, Illinois; and the American Anorexia/Bulimia Association, or AA/BA, now located in New York City. (See Appendix B.)

Slowly, the medical, psychiatric, and professional psychotherapy associations began to gear up with research studies and treatment programs to deal with this "new" disease—now an epidemic (one out of every two hundred and fifty girls ages eleven to twenty-two).

Some of these groups make referral to practitioners, local or national, who are experienced and specialize in eating disorders. Other groups provide self-help groups, often led by recovered victims of eating disorders. Parents' groups, formed in order to share their experience, advise and generally support each other. While some of these self-help groups are still going strong, others have disappeared as the professional medical and psychological establishments make greater commitments to help victims of the disease.

Self-help groups share similarities with alcoholic abuse groups, which sprang up for the same reasons. They are free of charge, they are anonymous, they are a safe introduction to help, no pressure is put on them the way psychotherapy "spotlights" the patient. They may also serve as a valuable adjunct to individual therapy.

The drawbacks are that such groups may comprise people of varying ages and diagnoses, and individuals may feel lost (along with their problems) in these "unscreened" groups.

Nevertheless, there is value in all treatment styles, when they are matched with the appropriate patient, client, or member of the eating-disordered population.

GRETA

Greta was twenty-three years old, five foot seven inches tall, and weighed eighty-two pounds. She sought treatment voluntarily, complaining of depression and the frequent arguments she had with her father over her weight and appearance. She had long, thinning brown hair in a braid. Though her face was skull-like in appearance, I could see that at a normal weight she was attractive. She brought in photos of herself at her normal, slim weight of one hundred and twenty-five pounds. She depreciated herself as fat in the pictures, though she was clearly pretty, with a well-proportioned figure. She complained about anxiety and not being able to sleep. I explained to her that these complaints were intensified, if not outright created, by her low weight and state of malnutrition. At the end of the session she asked if she could be in treatment with me. I said that I was willing to treat her if I—not she—remained in charge. She agreed.

After two sessions in the office, it was clear that Greta wasn't gaining any weight and was probably losing. She called to cancel the third session because her internist (an associate of mine) felt that she was too endangered to be treated outside a hospital. She also said that she believed she was too weak to come to the office anyway.

Later that afternoon, I received a call from the chief of psychiatry at the hospital to which she was admitted. He told me that Greta wasn't cooperating with the internists and had stated that if they treated her with central venous feeding (IV fluids), that she would sue them. Her weight had dropped to seventy-two pounds and her blood tests revealed that her heart, liver, and kidneys were beginning to fail; in other words, she was in imminent danger of dying. He told me that unless I could talk Greta into cooperating, they would have her certified as psychiatrically incompetent and would then continue their medical treatment to save her life without her permission.

I left for the hospital after office hours, taking with me a one-pound mylar mirror, four feet long. When I arrived at Greta's room, I was shocked. She was wearing a hospital gown which revealed that she was nothing but a skeleton covered with skin and veins, visible all over the surface of her skin. I immediately understood the psychiatrist's sense of urgency. In my näiveté I held up the mirror at the foot of the bed, expecting her to be shocked by her own appearance, the way I was. Greta laconically responded to her mirror image with "I think I look okay. I'm sure you mean well, but you're mistaken, just like the doctors here. I don't look too thin nor is my weight too low."

I put the mirror down. "If you don't agree to the medical measures necessary to save your life . . ." The phone rang. Greta reached for the handset, dragging it across the pillow toward her ear. She no longer had the strength to lift it. She told her father on the phone that she was feeling okay but the doctors were too worried and she didn't know what they would do to her. Then she hung up. I pointed out that she could not lift the phone, that she had no strength, that her heart, liver, and kidneys were all failing, that she was dying. She responded with, "I know you mean well but I'm feeling fine."

Well, so much for Mr. Nice Guy. "If you do not cooperate with the staff," I said much more firmly, "they will commit you, and you will not own your body for sixty days. The only way you can preserve your own dignity at this point is by cooperating as a voluntary patient rather than a committed patient."

Her languid look changed immediately. "I'm scared. I don't want them to make me fat!"

"Right now our major concern is to stop you from dying. We can argue cosmetic taste later." Noting her passivity and not wanting my patient committed, which somehow would make me feel like a failure, I picked her up and put her on a gurney at a right angle to her bed. Her head fell back against my hand, supporting her back, with the force of a bowling ball. She had no neck muscles left! I realized that I was carrying a virtual corpse. I put her on the rolling stretcher and headed for the unit that would start the necessary fluids to stop her from dying.

Greta's case had a healthy ending. She regained her weight, mostly through hyperalimentation (pumping a large number of nutritional calories through her jugular vein for weeks at a time). Once she had gained the weight, she maintained it by eating foods prescribed by the hospital dietitian.

She is an example of the most aggressive treatment necessary with anorexia—a treatment prohibited (due to the number of "bed days" involved) by most of today's insurance allowances. Greta was hospitalized for eighteen weeks. She continued to maintain her weight as an outpatient in individual psychotherapy. She was followed up for three additional years.

AINSLEY

Ainsley was twelve years old when she came into treatment. She was four foot nine and weighed fifty-eight pounds. She had started losing weight at seventy-eight pounds. She was not vomiting or taking laxatives, though she was exercising vigorously in her bedroom and severely restricting her food intake. She was probably eating no more than four hundred calories a day.

Ainsley had been seen frequently by her pediatrician, who was knowledgeable about anorexia. He had explained to Ainsley's mother that while he could place her in the pediatric/adolescent unit at his hospital, since she would be the youngest of the adolescent group, he was worried that she would be the most impressionable and learn additional eating disordered behaviors from the teens in the program. If he placed her on the unit with the younger children, he would had to have her fed intravenously to justify her staying in the hospital since there was no eating disorder program for pre-teens. He hoped that she could find a therapist she could trust and work with.

Ainsley was a shy, sullen child, who communicated with facial gestures (usually negative) rather than with words. At home, her mother explained, "It's as if Ainsley demands us to read her mind about her desires and dislikes. She speaks in a low voice, and her sentences are brief—usually just responses to our questions. She initiates very little conversation at home. She had one friend at school who moved away last year. Now she seems to have no friends at all."

Ainsley's weight had plummeted twenty pounds, but her physician still believed that she would do better with outpatient therapy unless a medical emergency occurred. In addition, he recommended that both Ainsley's parents see a second therapist who would advise them and coach them on restructuring their postures, demands, and limits to facilitate her giving up her anorexic behavior. In effect, they would create some of the hospital structure at home. Ainsley's parents had little resistance to restructuring the family system, with the support of the therapist, and her weight losing stopped within several weeks, followed by a period of stabilization. Finally, she began to achieve a $1^{1}/_{2}$- to 2-pound gain a week until she reached her goal weight.

Her other personality problems and issues took much longer to resolve than the loss of weight, as they usually do, but Ainsley stayed in therapy for two years after her goal weight was achieved.

MARGO

Margo had been sent home from college following a twenty-five-pound weight loss which left her emaciated. The college had attempted to help her with a counselor from Student Services, but there was no stopping her downward slide, despite threats of expulsion from the school, as well as offers of additional help if she "cooperated" with the school's demand that she turn around her weight-losing pattern.

Margo had been a freshman from late August to early December, when she was expelled from the college. She was what I term the "stateless citizen anorexic." She had no school to go to, her appearance denied her the possibility of getting jobs available to high school graduates, and all her friends had left town for other colleges at the same time she did but had not returned, so she had no friends.

Her medical examination was normal except for her weight and blood pressure—even emaciated anorexics can have mostly normal blood and organ functions; that doesn't mean that they are safe, however. The family's psychiatric hospital insurance allowed for twenty days' coverage; after that, the family would have to pay $700 per day out of pocket, which they could not afford.

Margo was sent to a local therapist for individual psychotherapy, as well as to a day program where she spent four hours (much less expensive than a hospital) and she joined an eating disorder support group, which was free.

Although most of Margo's day reinforced the idea that she had an eating disorder identity, it did not support the disorder. Without these three treatments she would have nothing but empty time to replace her days, formerly occupied by college attendance, which would drive her into further obsessionality and illness. This would also increase the worry, tension, anger, and divisiveness within the family, perhaps causing her younger sister and brother to feel jealous of the attention Margo was receiving.

Margo's parents were both working very hard full time and resented the loss of college tuition Margo's illness had cost them — in addition to the cost of two of the three treatments she was receiving. They did not have the time, money, or inclination to "give up" more than Margo's illness had cost them, so they did not enter a couples' therapy or support group.

Margo's progress varied between periods of recovering to her normal weight and losing weight and then regaining it.

JENNY

Jenny was twenty-three years old, graduated from college, lived alone in an apartment paid for by her parents. She had been anorexic for four years but not endangered medically. She had become severely rigid in her daily routines to the point where she could be diagnosed as obsessive-compulsive. As with other reclusive obsessive-compulsive disorder sufferers, her life became one ritual followed by another, from waking up, measuring her steps to the bathroom, picking up the toothbrush with her left hand, robotically transferring it to her right hand, counting the number of strokes each area of her mouth received, counting the number of times she stroked the bristles with her thumb under the running water to clean them, and so on through the day. Dressing and eating were done with the same lock-step precision. Indeed, Jenny had no time to go out of the apartment except for food shopping. She had little interaction with others, and no emotional connection with anyone that might influence her in any way.

She had traversed all four stages of anorexia with no interference by anyone at college or afterward. She *was* unhappy with her vegetative existence and called me for an appointment. I told her that I felt that she would need one significant person (to begin with) to compete with her illnesses and her lifestyle, and that she would have to come to individual psychotherapy from three to five days a week. Her parents could afford this as they could afford keeping her out of their sight in her own apartment. So we began.

Jenny did not make eye contact with me for nearly a year. I became a surrogate parent and began to tell her how I wanted her to manage her life. I scolded her when she didn't follow my recommendations; she argued intensely with me and accused me of taking advantage of my "power" over her: "You know that you are the only person I talk to every day!" I used this extraordinary bond that was developing to compete with her compulsive rules.

Very gradually, over five years, Jenny transferred her emotional priorities from the intrapersonal (within her own head only) to the interpersonal, between us. For those of you who wonder how such a therapeutic relationship ever ends, since it is a reparenting relationship, remember that healthy children outgrow their desire to be treated like children or adolescents and eventually move out. The therapeutically reparented patient "grows up" in therapy and "moves out" also. I haven't heard from Jenny for several years, but I do get holiday greeting cards with pictures of her growing family. We will see more of Jenny in chapter 12.

Behavior Modification — The Least Personal Treatment

Most behavior modification treatments are programs that are based on reward and punishment (for weight gain and eating) and are carried out in hospital settings.

On the surface, behavior modification is coercive behavior to produce compliant behavior by the patient. When this is truly all the program offers, the patient will outwardly comply, grudgingly, then she will lose the weight coerced upon her as soon as she is discharged from the hospital. This appears to be an exercise in futility, though often it may be temporarily successful in saving someone's life or disrupting a destructive pattern at its most energetic. So, it is still a valuable tool.

At its most successful, an inpatient behavioral modification program has other components to it: group therapy led by experienced leaders; individual therapy done by sensitive therapists; and the patient community meetings, which encourage better peer relationships in a safe setting. In successful programs (with low rates of relapse after discharge), the patient becomes attached to the entire program and her anorexic-obsessional patterns are overwhelmed by the external stimuli everyone around her represents. In effect, the program "drowns out" her habitual mental activities and rules, protecting her from her sick, isolated self. The power and consistency of the program are experienced as protective, even if she is afraid of others in the program.

One important dynamic must be present in this setting, however: what we call a "treatment alliance." This is a connection with one or more persons in the program, ideally including at least one staff member and perhaps one or several patients. The "alliance" refers to her seeing that person or those persons as trustworthy, likable, and consistent, while remaining powerful.

CAROL

Carol was sixteen when she entered a firmly structured behavioral modification program in an eating disorder unit at a psychiatric hospital. She had suffered a major weight loss of twenty-five pounds over a period of five months. Her parents didn't want to be too strict with her, but their sensitivity to her requests, which became demands as time went on, made them angry and terrified for their daughter's life. They "surrendered" their daughter to the hospital. As her father put it, "I hope you can stop her from dying . . . we can't."

Carol tested the program. She tried exercising by doing pushups in her room until she was discovered. She planned on vomiting until she found out someone would be listening when she used the bathroom. The door was always left ajar. Finally, she believed the program would overpower all her abilities to control her weight. She became frightened and continually called home, begging that she would behave if only she were allowed to go home and leave "this awful place." Her parents—feeling guilty and worried—called her outpatient therapist. He assured them that their best hope was to tell Carol that she could not expect to leave the hospital until she had reached her goal weight.

Carol cried continually on the phone and in the hospital unit as well. She spent days crying, until she began to talk to a psychiatric worker she felt close to. Next, she was talking in her group therapy sessions until other fears were being expressed—not just about food, weight, and homesickness, but about who she was, where she belonged, and how empty she felt. This was a turning point in her inpatient treatment. She surrendered her disordered behavior to the hospital's rules and her secret fears to others in the program, both patients and staff.

Carol would need outpatient treatment for a long period of time in order to overcome her difficulty with trust and to substitute dependency for illness.

Obviously, many considerations are involved in deciding which kind of treatment will be successful in helping a victim overcome anorexia nervosa. Often treatments must be changed as the patient's health and circumstances improve or deteriorate. Matching the mode of treatment to the patient's current situation is the major challenge in evaluating and prescribing treatment. All of the treatments I have described here are helpful to different patients in different stages of the illness. Medication as a possible adjunct to each of these modes is discussed in later chapters, as well as in Appendix A.

12

TRANSFERENCE
AND CREATING AN ALLIANCE
FOR TREATMENT

Transference

POPULAR myths about psychotherapy suggest that most cures rely on the discovery of some hidden mental secret, stored deep within the unconscious. Until recently, the importance of the relationship between patient and therapist has been largely overlooked. Early theoreticians like Wilhelm Reich, who emphasized the patient-therapist relationship in his book, *The Analysis of Transference* (1949), are in the minority, possibly because therapists are reticent in acknowledging the role their own personalities play in the recovery of their patients.

As children, we all are attuned to the personalities as well as the emotional needs of the people closest to us. Throughout our lives, we unknowingly form generalizations about other people as well, based on these early sets of ideas. These personality models can be based on a parent, an older sibling, or grandparents, depending on who were the most important figures throughout childhood. We usually don't apply these generalities to the person who does our dry cleaning, the grocer, or the paperboy. Such generalizations only come into play when a person becomes important to us.

At this point, we transfer onto new people the collection of feelings and expectations we have carried with us since early childhood. For example, if a child's father has a volatile temper, triggered unpredictably and without apparent provocation, that child will grow to become fearful throughout life that anyone she becomes close to will, without warning, strike out verbally or physically. This is her *transferential expectation*, learned from her relationship with her father.

There are as many transferential expectations as there are relationship styles between parent and child. I have mentioned the importance of a parent-child relationship that is based on trust, attachment, and dependency. The experience of this type of relationship, when transferred to a new significant other, can result in the expectation of the same, positive, healthy qualities from the new person. If these expectations are reciprocated by the new person, a rich relationship can develop.

If one's childhood relationship with a parent is a negative experience—incorporating mistrust, nondependability, and hostile attachment rather than trustworthiness, dependency, and positive attachment—then one will transfer the same negative expectations one has learned as a child to new important relationships later on. When this happens, the expectations either destroy the relationship, or create a dysfunctional relationship parallel to the person's original parent-child relationship.

Amongst anorexics, we see the recurrence of a similar parent-child relationship with at least one parent (usually but not always the mother). It is common for an anorexic to believe that her primary caregiver is intimidated by her, and has always been intimidated by her, especially when she was a child. Consequently, she expects that any adult who will ever play a significant role in her life will be intimidated by her, and will be needy of whatever support she can offer them. She comes into a relationship expecting the other person to fail to be a substantial, dependable, and emotional resource in her own time of need. These feelings leave her contemptuous and cynical of the people in her life, for what she sees as their inability to be trusted.

When someone with anorexia nervosa enters into treatment, she does so not as a patient, but as an investigator of the therapist's character. And as an investigator, she is anything but partial. She is searching for signs that would confirm the transferential expectation she learned in her relationship with a parent. She hopes to find anything that would betray her therapist as being insensitive (the inattentive or disengaged parent) or as being needy of her strength (the dependent parent).

Although it is easier to spot insensitivity, signs of neediness must be elicited. In therapy, the anorexic can satisfy this transferential expectation if she can prove to herself that her therapist needs her approval, her acceptance. She might go about this by rejecting the therapist, responding to him or her with silence, distance, indifference.

My task as a therapist is to thwart the patient's attempts to construe me as either insensitive or needy. If I were to react personally to a patient's attempts at rejecting me, either by behaving equally as indifferently to her as she acts toward me, or by responding to her resistance to my help with my own hurt feelings, I would prove to her that I was just like every other adult who had failed her. By not allowing myself to be manipulated, I come across as someone who is not only there to help her but who needs neither her support, her approval, nor her perfection to lead a fulfilled life. In other words, she is able to see me in a way that she has never thought of anyone: *dependable*. This is a foundation upon which she can build her trust in me. As a result, we can begin to form a treatment alliance in which our mutual interest is to eradicate the behavior that rules her life and makes her miserable.

Forming a treatment alliance is not easy. Because the alliance the anorexic needs to form with her therapist in order to realize change is unfamiliar to her, it is frightening. At the same time, however, while she feels frightened, the prospect of having such a rela-

tionship appeals to her secret wish to depend upon and trust someone—a wish that she consciously denies herself in order to avoid
what she perceives as an inevitable disappointment. The will to sup-
press her need to have someone to trust is strong, and I am continually working against her resistance in a manner that is outside the
realm of her transferential expectations.

I use the term "resistance" to refer to an unconscious defensive
behavior that protects the anorexic from what she expects of others
based on her personal history. This defense mechanism keeps her
emotionally guarded and cynical. Resistance is steeped in the
patient's inability to understand how her past can bias her outlook
on a new relationship before it even starts.

Overcoming Resistance with a Nurturant-
Authoritative Approach

If a child senses that her parent is intimidated by her, she feels she
can't depend on that parent. Although her ability to intimidate her
parent may instill in her a superficial sense of power, its primary
impact is the feeling that the parent has abandoned her. If an adult
shows signs of being intimidated by his or her own child, becoming
hurt and saddened when a small child acts out, or reacting with
anger as if a child's temper tantrums pose a threat to the adult, the
child senses that she is the most powerful figure in her world.
Because she is made to feel that the fate of her parents' happiness
or unhappiness (as the case may be) lies in her hands, she learns
that she cannot depend on anyone as a stable source of support and
authority. She learns to feel that she is the only person who can
make herself feel safe.

This is where resistance is formed. She must keep herself guarded and invulnerable to others, for if, as a child, her own parents
failed to be dependable, then who could she ever trust? In extreme
cases, it is common to find that the anorexic actually parented one
of her own parents from a very young age. Not only was she

deprived of the experience of having her own emotional needs met, but she took on the job of parenting one or the other parent, of taking care of them.

The child who was never made to feel safe and secure, the child who was depended upon rather than allowed her own dependencies, carries these unrequited needs into adolescence and then adulthood. She resents her need to depend on someone because she was taught that it will never be met. In fact, she is frightened by the prospect that she has emotional needs, after having to deny them for so long. She tells herself that this is weakness, and to stop hoping that her needs will ever be met.

The therapist who, by his or her demeanor, suggests that these wishes for dependency and guidance can be met in the therapeutic relationship, is a threat to her. The opportunity to have someone she can trust (something she deeply longs for) weakens her defenses, evokes hope, and makes her vulnerable.

It is useful for a therapist to explain this at the beginning of therapy, even as early as the first session. The unconscious cannot be fooled or tricked, but it can be disarmed of its resistance by making clear what the therapeutic relationship and process involve. I always warn someone who has come to see me for a consultation, as was the case with Jenny (see chapter 11).

"It will be very difficult for you to be in treatment with me."

"Why?"

"Because you won't know who to be when you're talking to me. You're used to being the caregiver, the congenial, confident exterior, or the tyrant. What you don't know is how to receive help."

Oftentimes the patient reacts with an unpleasant expression at the words "help," "receive," or both.

"Your reaction suggests that within five or six weeks you'll want to stop keeping your appointments, cancel them in advance, or quit therapy."

"Why should I want to do that?"

"Because that Little Jenny inside you who has always wished for someone to depend on, and has always been stifled by your pessimism, will begin to emerge. First you will become louder, and then you will no longer be able to stifle her at all. You will become upset with me, and with therapy, for weakening you and making Little Jenny stronger. I will make it difficult for you to deny your wish for dependency by proving myself to be a person you can depend on."

Jenny's eyes welled up as I spoke about the path ahead.

"Do you feel that sadness right now? The reason your eyes are welling up with tears and you're even considering crying is that I made Little Jenny louder."

The tears ran freely down Jenny's face as she stared at the floor.

"Those are precious tears because you're directing them to someone else, not an empty room. They will restore you. That is one way you can take something from me, receive something; you'll have someone who will listen."

Jenny began to talk through her crying. "I don't know what I'm supposed to say. I hate this. I always know what to say. You're not my father. Some day this will be over and I won't see you anymore. Why should I talk to you about me just so it'll tear me up when I'm finished with therapy? It's crazy. I can't go home with you. It's so artificial."

"If you break your leg, you need a cast and a crutch. Both of these are artificial and temporary needs that must be filled so your leg can heal. Then your leg heals and you don't need a cast and a crutch. When the leg heals, you outgrow them."

"But a relationship is different. You don't just outgrow it!"

"A young child is very dependent on her parents to guide her and to make her feel safe and protected. Parents are the most important people in a child's life. If a child is made to feel that she can trust her parents, that they are dependable and a reliable source of care, then she can enjoy the shelter they have created with their love and discipline. A child needs the boundaries of this shelter, otherwise she would feel unprotected in an infinitely large world.

"If these needs are met in childhood, this dependency lessens through the years—into adolescence and adulthood—as she becomes able to face more and more of the world without their help. She outgrows the needs of a child, and as an adult, her attachment to her parents is based more on love and appreciation than on need.

"If these needs aren't met, as yours were not, they never go away. You still have the need for someone to make you feel safe in this world, and because you resent that need and fear that it will never go away, you hide from it, in your anorexic symptoms."

Jenny looked skeptical: "Are you saying that *you* can create a parentlike relationship with me, get those needs satisfied, and I can outgrow you? I find that hard to believe."

"I told you earlier that it will be hard for you to be in treatment with me. The first thing you'll have to do is to take the risk that the idea you've just scoffed at is true. If you don't, you'll always have Little Jenny to contend with and you'll need your symptoms to shut her up."

"Risk, huh?" she said, smiling. "That's an interesting way of looking at it. Maybe I'll try it." And with a mock-serious look she added, "You better be right."

"I still think that you'll want to quit after the first few months."

"Jeeez. I said I'll try it. Why are you trying to sabotage this case before it even starts?"

"I just want you to remember that when you're tempted not to show up for an appointment, you have to make yourself fight your resistance and show up anyway."

"Okay, okay, point made. You're right. It's already hard to be in treatment with you."

"Do you want me to schedule regular appointments for you?"

Her answer was labored and slow, "Yeah—I guess so."

"Does that mean 'Yes'?"

"I guess so."

"There is 'Yes' and any other answer is 'Not Yes.' "

"Okay! *Yes.*"

Jenny and I had begun the struggle that would eventually help her to overcome her symptoms and confront their causes, the struggle that told her, during the first meeting, that I was substantial (or wouldn't "flake out on her," as she might have said), and that she was not too much trouble for me.

In this struggle which shapes the course of therapy, there is a delicate balance between nurturing and authoritative behavior. If I err on the side of being all-nurturing and lack authority, and the ability to confront her, Jenny will become contemptuous of me for failing to follow through on my offer to be dependable. She will feel abandoned and lose the ability to make herself trust me in spite of her resistance. On the other hand, if I am all-authoritative—powerful but not caring—Jenny will disconnect from me. Even if she outwardly complies because she is intimidated by my authority, she will not feel connected. That emotional connection provides us with the leverage that is essential for helping Jenny change.

That first session was like a test drive for Jenny; she was trying out what it would be like to be in treatment. No therapist should be lulled into a sense of security after a successful first encounter with a patient. Trust and connection don't develop for some time. The development of this kind of therapeutic relationship is in competition with the resistance that Jenny's entire life was based on before she met me. All I could do in that first meeting was try to evoke some hope and curiosity, both of which would create conflict with Jenny's cynicism. In her resistance, no doubt, she would attempt to devalue me almost as soon as she left the office.

Creating an Alliance

During the initial period of therapy—the first two months—it is desirable to meet twice a week so that the patient is never more than three days away from reinforcement of the idea that she now has someone she can trust. I am continuously competing with the anorexic's past learning. If we consistently forego too many days without a session, her resistance will have time to mobilize so that each session will be like starting from square one. If the sessions are close together, they build on each other and mistrust has a smaller window in which to develop.

Suppose there are no financial limitations (and there usually are), the frequency of meetings is determined by the amount of time that has elapsed since the onset of the anorexia, as well as the degree to which the patient has become emotionally separated from other people. In some cases, this could mean as many as five sessions a week for some chronically ill patients, and as few as the minimum (once a week) for others.

Realistically, one to two sessions per week is all that most individuals and families can afford, if that. The burden is then on the therapist to keep alert to every nuance in the progression of his or her relationship with the patient. These observations must be continually interpreted for and explained to the patient, for example:

Jenny did not make eye contact with me for the first year of treatment. She did, however, steal the occasional glance at me, apparently in an effort to prepare herself for the time when she could look at me while she talked about herself in therapy. I noticed one of these glances.

"I notice that you haven't made eye contact with me in the two months that we have been meeting."

"I just can't do that yet. It's too personal. It's easier for me to make eye contact with people who aren't important."

"I thought I saw you looking at me for a brief instant a minute ago, and that was a change."

"Maybe."

"Perhaps you're becoming a little safer here."

"I'm not 'safe' anywhere."

"I'm sure you haven't been."

"But you're so sure that I will be, huh?"

"Yes, I suppose I am."

"You're pretty sure of yourself. I guess you have a pretty big ego."

"I'm pretty sure that you'll become safer here."

"You're pretty cocky, aren't you?"

"Sometimes you can be a brat."

"You can't call me a brat—you're my therapist! Therapists can't call their patients brats!" She kicked the floor several times.

"I guess if you are going to act like a brat, I'll have to identify that. It doesn't mean that I don't like you, or that our relationship is in jeopardy. It just means that you're showing me a part of you that you could never show at home with your parents because you were afraid of their reaction."

Jenny's transference was very strong. She was recently released from the hospital where she had been put when her weight dropped to a dangerous low. The hospital designated her prognosis as "fair"—not very optimistic. She was living alone in an extra apartment her parents kept. I was seeing her five days a week. She told me in no uncertain terms, "You are the only person I talk to every day."

This can have pitfalls as well as advantages. Five sessions a week can intensify a patient's transferential feelings until the therapy becomes a battleground where the therapist is literally perceived as the patient's parents. Such a climate can be helpful because more can be accomplished sooner. However, such an intense level of interaction can also be a threat to the boundaries of the patient-therapist relationship. Jenny had a strict sense of boundaries instilled in her from her "distant and proper" relationship with her parents, thus making it less of a risk to see her so often. A patient with a weaker sense of boundaries should not be seen more than twice a week.

Boundaries and Dependency

The first treatment issue the therapist has to deal with is to figure out how to maintain his or her own boundaries and not become anxious, while allowing the patient to become emotionally close. Physical contact, even a pat on the back by the therapist, might invite a breakdown of boundaries on both sides of the patient-therapist relationship. This possibility must be considered by the therapist.

In the past, most clinical training explained how to cope with patients' hostility rather than the issue of their potential for attachment. As therapy styles move further away from the strict rules of psychoanalysis (where the therapist's role is passive and primarily consists of listening), they have become more interactive, with the therapist doing more talking. Because, in this type of interactive relationship, the therapist is more involved in the life of his patient, he is more responsible for the patient's reaction to him than if he were simply doing a lot of listening.

When we, as therapists, talk to our patients and initiate a relationship, we take a risk. We enter into an interpersonal arena with the patient. This is not a task for the fainthearted therapist. Yet without such intense involvement in the psychotherapy, the therapist is not in a position to compete with the anorexia—a disease that, for the patient, has become a way of life, and the only way of living.

The question then becomes: What happens to this intensive therapeutic relationship, and the anorexic's dependency on her therapist, when it is time to wind down and end treatment? Therapists have asked me this question because they fear that if they allow their patients to become dependent on them, it may not be a temporary part of the healing process, but evolve into a lifetime attachment. I assure them that if they allow the patient to "grow up" in therapy, they will see several changes in the intensity of the patient's dependence.

Initially, the dependency deepens. After the first year or two, it levels off, and then decreases until the developmental issues (that exist because the needs were never met in childhood) of trust, attachment, identity, intimacy, and sexuality are successfully addressed. When this happens, the patient no longer needs the crutch and cast, and does in fact begin to grow out of the patient-therapist relationship. At that point she usually indicates a desire to decrease the frequency of sessions, or to begin discussing a termination date.

The time frame for the recovery process varies with each patient. Major factors in this variation are the mental health and emotional resourcefulness of the patient's family, as well as any genetic predispositions or biochemical disturbances that can affect depression or anxiety. Regardless of these factors, the time necessary for recovery almost always lies outside the timetables created by HMOs for which they will provide monetary reimbursement.

The daunting nature of the task at hand, the prospect of challenging the anorexia head-on and grappling with all of its demons, may be one reason why we have such poor recovery statistics. In this day and age, we can't even imagine the oncologist who would balk at the detection of cancer in a patient, too intimidated by the disease to proceed with treatment. In the case of anorexia nervosa, however, practitioners are oftentimes reluctant to confront the reality of this powerful disease and take the steps necessary to realize a cure. The statistics for probable recovery range from 25 to 35 percent, according to the National Association of Anorexia Nervosa and Associated Disorders. The relatively new twelve-step approach declares that a victim of the disease remains a recovering anorexic for life.

I see 85 to 90 percent of my patients recover. I have a desk drawer full of baby pictures sent to me by new mothers who were, at one time, skinny teenage patients of mine.

When parents raise a child, the child's life is completely dependent upon them. This dependency gradually diminishes in the healthy son or daughter until he or she is able to leave the parents' home. I offer this summary of healthy parenting as a parallel for my treatment relationship with victims of anorexia nervosa (and indeed of most psychological disorders).

Anorexia nervosa is a disorder whose predisposition develops in childhood or early adolescence. There can be no doubt that treating it, compensating for it, and the psychological rebuilding necessary to heal it, all require a large commitment of time, energy, and skill from everyone involved.

13

PARENTS AND REPARENTING

WOULD like to address the ways parents can support therapeutic change to help their children recover from this stubborn disorder. Most anorexics' family systems have characteristic relationships that foster a continuation of the disorder. The members involved unknowingly cooperate with each other to prevent change, even if they all agree that change is needed. Before we look at case study illustrations of successful changes in family systems, I want to discuss families who have fallen into certain pitfalls.

Some Pitfalls to Therapeutic Family Change

Sometimes we all know what is the correct way to do something, but we sabotage ourselves from doing it, whether or not we are aware of the sabotage.

DOROTHY AND ANNE

Dorothy's daughter Anne developed anorexia at the age of fourteen.

Dorothy was married to George, who was a retired businessman. They had one other child, a son. George had many interests; esoteric hobbies, mainly the study of antiquities and fieldwork in archeology. This often took him away from home for periods of weeks or longer. Dorothy was a clinical psychologist. The son, now aged twenty-three, lived near his former college, quite a distance away. Also living with the family was Carmen, a seventeen-year-old girl whose family had been killed in an auto accident.

Dorothy was very close to her own mother, who lived with her father a block away. Dorothy was involved in community volunteer projects, and also focused on the two girls who lived with her. At the time her daughter developed anorexia, Dorothy seemed very concerned with her daughter. She observed her eating and exercising, and often asked her how much she weighed. The first time they came in—Dorothy, George, and Anne—one could not miss the annoyed, contemptuous tone in Anne's voice and the way she rolled her eyes each time her mother spoke. Equally obvious was Dorothy's fear of displeasing her daughter as she finished every sentence with a smile, a compliment about Anne, and often a request that Anne verify what her mother had just said—"Isn't that right, dear?" George, on the other hand, was continually chiding his wife for letting her daughter dominate her. She would answer back with, "George thinks you can solve any problem with a command. That's how he ran his business. It's certainly not the way one operates in the field of psychology."

"Well, I don't see Anne stopping losing weight in response to all your 'understanding,' " her husband retorted. "It goes further," he continued. "This woman is practically a slave to her daughter. She will do anything for her—buy her anything, take her anywhere. I don't think that she ever says no to Anne."

Anne interjected, "She says no to me plenty. You're just never home when it happens. Sometimes it feels like you're never home. I can't understand why you even care," voicing a grievance in support of her mother.

Anne had an interesting position in her family system. When her father was not around or involved in an issue she and her mother discussed, she was hostile and disrespectful toward her mother. When her father argued with her mother about her, Anne would jump to her mother's defense. When other issues than Anne arose, she sided with her father and the mother was outnumbered two to one.

Dorothy was a bright, psychologically educated woman, who presented rational explanations for her accommodating behavior toward Anne: Anne was the youngest; her brother who she adored had moved out on her (and the family); and Anne had accepted Carmen living with them with no hostility nor jealousy. Dorothy portrayed Anne as deprived compared to her sibling and Carmen, and almost a martyr in her mind, who needed compensation.

Anne clenched her jaw, stared straight ahead at no one, clearly feeling righteous and good about this defense of her.

I asked Anne, "How do you feel about what your mother just said about the situation?"

Anne's jaw slackened; her eyes lost their righteous intensity. She shrugged. "I don't think about that stuff much. I guess it's right."

I continued, "Do you feel like the most deprived member of the family, do you feel gypped?"

"I don't know if I feel gypped, but I don't agree with all those other things my father said about me, either. I don't think it's fair to call her [Dorothy] my slave and make me sound like some sort of monster."

I looked around at the three of them. "We have three descriptions of three people, none of which corroborate the other two. None of you see your relationships the same."

I waited.

George just shook his head, staring down at the floor.

Dorothy monitored her daughter until Anne's breathing became rapid. Then Dorothy broke the silence. "Many families have multiple points of view. It is rare that all members of the family see their family the same way. I don't think there's anything unusual here. I see this in my own work with families."

I looked at Dorothy. "Dorothy, do you see anything unusual or problematic in your family? George has voiced his opinion, and while you disagreed and defended your posture toward Anne, it doesn't seem that you've had your say about problems that exist in relationships between the three of you, or even problems that may include your son or Carmen, though they're not here."

Dorothy looked surprised. "I don't believe in looking on the negative side of things. None of us is perfect and none of us is a monster. George and I disagree somewhat about how Anne should be treated, but that's not serious."

"If you and George are polarized over Anne, which you seem to downplay, would that polarization possibly contribute to Anne's problems?"

"If I knew the answer to that, I guess we wouldn't be here, would we?" She smiled at me.

"Sometimes members of a family know what's wrong and feel too uncomfortable to change their own role in it." I looked around the room signaling that I wasn't singling out Dorothy.

In subsequent sessions, additional family conflicts emerged. Dorothy protested her retired husband's "hobby," which took him away from the house, leaving her to do all of the parenting while offering her no support at all when he traveled around the world being a "dilettante archeologist"—the eternal tourist, leaving her to do all the "real" work of running a family. After saying this, she burst into tears and apologized to her husband for hurting his feelings, and to her daughter for making her sound like a burden. She vowed such an outburst would never happen again and blamed it on other pressures at work.

Meanwhile, Anne continued to lose weight. She offered little meaningful talk in her individual sessions and claimed that her health, and relationships at home, were fine.

Anne's weight dropped to seventy-nine pounds at a height of five foot seven. I called her home, after speaking with her pediatrician who indicated that she was technically "in good health," meaning she had no abnormal blood or organ functions. Neither of us was comfortable allowing her to remain an outpatient: she should be hospitalized before she became an emergency or worse.

Dorothy seemed shocked at the weight loss and defended her daughter's eating, at least when her daughter was eating in her presence. She was horrified at the idea of putting Anne in a medical hospital and made no reference to the pediatrician's concerns or my own about her daughter's situation. Nevertheless, she agreed to take Anne to the community hospital where I would continue seeing her as a "visiting psychotherapist" co-treating Anne with a psychiatrist and a gastroenterologist.

I routinely stopped at the nurses' station on my way to a patient's room. I would read the chart notes and have informal discussions with the floor nurses about the patient's progress.

The first time I went to see Anne, the nurses on the unit, who knew me from previous hospitalizations, asked me to step into their private conference room. I knew this couldn't be good news. As we sat around in a circle of chairs and couches, the head nurse spoke first.

Anne had been hiding food under her bed and flushing what she could down the toilet. She was put on a nasogastric tube to prevent her from losing more weight (she had lost a pound in the hospital). They found out she had been disconnecting the tube and letting the fluids run into a pitcher, which she would pour down the toilet. This time she had miscalculated: the liquid nutrition bag was emptied two hours early. Anne claimed to know nothing about it.

She was transferred to a room with a television camera and her bathroom was locked. She had to ring for a nurse when she wanted to go to the bathroom and the nurse would observe her there.

When her mother heard about this "invasion of her daughter's privacy" via a complaint from Anne, she left work immediately and went to the hospital to protest. The head nurse told her about

Anne's sabotaging her own treatment, but Dorothy made it clear that she did not believe this and hadn't knowingly put her daughter into a "prison" for treatment. Anne asked her mother to bring her a pizza for dinner to prove the nurses' allegations wrong. Dorothy drove thirty miles to bring Anne the pizza from the specific restaurant she requested.

The nurse on duty told Dorothy that Anne should only be eating what the dietician selected in cooperation with Anne. Dorothy replied that she would consider signing her daughter out of the hospital if some flexibility was not shown. After all, Anne was there to gain weight. "Why shouldn't she be allowed to eat something as fattening as pizza?"

The nurse retreated and made a chart note of the incident, as well as other incidents such as Dorothy breaking rules by visiting her daughter four to five times a day, smuggling food into her room, and in general indicating to Anne, who had only gained two pounds in three weeks, that she would be going home soon. Dorothy also alluded to her unhappiness with the nursing staff and her daughter's general hospital care.

The nursing staff were antagonized by what they described as Dorothy's attitude that they were baby-sitters, that they should try to go along with Anne and her breach of the rules set up as treatment.

After four weeks, Anne was discharged from the hospital having gained three pounds. A gain of two pounds per week would have been optimal. The hospital Utilization and Review Committee deemed further hospitalization of Anne at this point nonproductive and unnecessary.

Anne returned to my office after canceling her first appointment. Her posture was distantly pleasant and casual. It was clear there was no therapeutic alliance between us. When we had discussed whether she wanted to continue in therapy, Anne requested that she not schedule any appointment in advance at this time. She would call me if she wanted to return to treatment.

Three months later, Dorothy called me to indicate that Anne was considered endangered by her low weight again and she wanted my opinion as to which of two hospitals I considered more suitable for her daughter. She sounded upset and hopeless, but I could hear that the hopelessness was just as much about changing her relationship with her daughter as about her daughter's recovery.

For the next two years, like many other girls with anorexia, Anne was in and out of several hospitals at four-month intervals and had seen three outpatient psychotherapists.

I called this section "Pitfalls." A major treatment focus in this case should have been the enmeshed relationship that existed between Anne and her mother, the reversal of dominance, where daughter dominated needy mother, and the lack of support the mother was getting from her husband, causing her to turn to her daughter for emotional support. The result was an unhealthy pact between mother and daughter whereby the daughter was the mother's support in exchange for the mother's support against all others who would interfere with Anne's anorexic behavior—which the daughter could rely on for security.

Not all cases are treatable. Some family systems allow the therapeutic intrusion; others don't. It is difficult for any family to invite a stranger into their most personal and private feelings toward each other.

GINA

Gina was seventeen years old, both anorexic and bulimic. Her parents were not familiar with psychotherapy, did not want to participate in any parent or family therapy, but believed that their daughter's illness should be treated. When they were told by their family doctor that part or all of the treatment involved psychotherapy, they brought her in "to be cured."

Gina showed up regularly for twice weekly appointments; she was very open and emotional about the way she felt about herself, her parents, and her poor social and academic standing at school.

One day in between appointments, Gina's mother called. Her voice was assertive but not hostile. "Steven, I want you to know that I can see how much my daughter likes you. I can also see that she is eating better and gaining weight. I want you to understand one thing. I am trusting you with my daughter's care, but remember, what's mine is mine, and Gina is *mine*. I don't want you to forget that."

I confess I was delighted with such straightforward talk. I enjoyed responding with, "Maureen, I don't want to become your daughter's parent and I bet you don't want to be her therapist."

"Well, you're right. I don't want your job. I hear enough from her as it is, but I wanted to make sure you understand how I feel."

"Then we have a deal. Gina remains your daughter and my patient."

"Steven, we have a deal," she said in a hoarse, friendly voice.

What could have become a pitfall became the slightest bump on the road to Gina's recovery, which was complete within two years.

Despite Maureen's worry or jealousy about losing her daughter's love, and her daughter's attachment to a therapist, she was so open about it that it didn't prevent Gina from developing a strong therapeutic alliance and attachment to me, which during the acute part of her illness remained intense and dependent. As she recovered from the acute phase of her illness, I could see Gina's alliance diminishing. She had her mother's emotional permission to be in therapy, with all the relationship complications that come with that. In time, Gina did what we want all our patients to do: recover from their illness, outgrow it, and outgrow the therapist as well. It usually settles into holiday greeting cards, often with marital announcements and later baby pictures.

RONNIE

Sometimes a parent is in too much conflict to "let go." I received a call one day from a woman with an assertive, no-nonsense style of speaking. "My daughter, Ronnie, has been diagnosed as having anorexia nervosa. I want to get her in treatment as soon as possible. I've read that the sooner this is treated, the quicker the recovery. She's fifteen, five foot three, and has gone from a hundred and twenty to ninety pounds. At first I was pleased. She weighed too much, anyway. I made a deal with her. She has a large nose. I told her I thought that she would look better if we "took a little off her nose" and to go with her new nose she could lose ten pounds. When she lost the ten pounds, I would schedule the surgery for her nose. She seemed to agree with me and began losing weight.

"When she reached a hundred and ten, I told her that was enough, or almost enough, anyway. But the weight loss increased instead of stopping. She was losing nearly three pounds a week now and she's down to ninety—but that was last week. I don't know what she weighs today. All of this took a little over three months. I hear kids have this for years. I think we caught it early so maybe this can be stopped quickly," she concluded.

Now it was my turn to talk. "I'm impressed by your ability to focus on problems and their solutions. I do think that three months is 'early detection' and often this gives the treatment a good prognosis. But before I can respond any further, we have to schedule an appointment with your daughter for an evaluation. I have to meet with her. When can she come in?"

"Well, she has a busy schedule, but we'll move it around. When do you have time available?"

For her first appointment, Ronnie came ten minutes early. I buzzed her in and told her over the intercom that I would be ten minutes. When she entered the office, she immediately greeted me with "I'm sorry I was early."

I responded, "That's what waiting rooms are for. Coming early is surely a virtue in contrast with coming late."

"I'm still sorry. I hope that I didn't disturb you or your last patient."

There was no consoling this self-effacing girl of fifteen. "Why don't you take a seat. I use the swivel chair; you can have the couch or the overstuffed chair."

"Would you prefer that I take one or the other?"

"No."

She looked around and chose the chair. I thought this was a remarkable contrast of submissiveness and self-effacement from a girl who was fighting off her world of parents, doctors, friends, and relatives all asking her to stop losing and start gaining weight. She had found her own way of saying no without seeing herself as defiant.

I asked her why she was sent to me. She replied, "My mother made it clear to me that I was 'tubby.' I even think she used that word, but I'm not sure. Then she told me that I needed a nose job, that my nose was unacceptable and should be altered. I suppose she wants some little 'button' between my eyes. I don't."

"Then you're satisfied with your appearance and you don't want anyone telling you how you should look?"

"No! I hate the way I look. I think I'm ugly."

"You've lost a lot of weight. Does that make you feel better about yourself?"

"When I was a hundred and twenty, I thought this would be a horrifyingly low weight. Even a hundred sounded too low. Now that I'm ninety, I'm tempted to play into the eighties. I don't feel too thin at this weight. One hundred pounds sounds like I'd be a blimp. It's all changed. But I'm really terrified to gain weight and at the same time I hate how it's hurting my mother . . . and father."

"Do you often displease, argue, or fight with them?"

"Only when the issue is going out at night or sleeping over at a friend's house. My mother always says no, although it's always at a girlfriend's house and it's not a party. I just think that most of her rules are designed to keep me close to her. I don't think she wants me to grow up, and that makes me so mad at her."

"Then do you defy her on these issues?"

"Hardly ever. It makes me feel too guilty. Then I find myself worrying about her being upset. It's crazy in a way. Whenever I get angry, I also feel sorry for her at the same time. The only thing that seems consistent is that I weigh too much and I'm ugly."

"Do you like that consistency—knowing you feel ugly, without the conflict when you feel angry at your mother?"

"I *am* ugly, so it's easy."

"You don't seem sad about this idea that you're ugly."

"Well, I'm not happy about it. You know, I have a beautiful sister. I'm often told by my mother that I could be as beautiful as my sister if I wanted to. So she thinks I'm ugly, too."

Ronnie kept her appointments twice a week for one month. During that time, she stopped losing weight and even gained two pounds. She had mentioned that her mother grumbled about Ronnie having two mothers and alluded to my being inconsistent with Ronnie. She also complained that she was being left out in the cold in terms of Ronnie's treatment.

Ronnie did not show up for her tenth appointment. I called the house and her mother said that Ronnie had left the house after an early dinner and she didn't know where she went. Ronnie did not return two calls I made to her. Her father answered the third call. I indicated that Ronnie had not been in contact with me for several weeks so I assumed she had dropped out of treatment and canceled her hours. Her father attempted to assure me that "She'll be back." I just asked him to convey that message to his daughter. He said that he would.

Two more weeks went by and still no contact from Ronnie. Subsequently, her mother called me and in the same assertive voice, as if she were taking me to task, stated, "We have to talk." I told her I thought that was a good idea but she would have to come in for an appointment. She suddenly sounded disappointed (apparently expecting me to hold an open-ended conversation with her on the phone) and somewhat anxious.

In our conference, I told her that I didn't think I could help her daughter directly. I told her that I believed her daughter didn't want a therapist but wanted her mother. I told her that I would like her to come in every week for awhile and we could talk and examine family issues, her relationship with her husband, the sisters' relationship, and her own relationship with Ronnie. She looked very surprised and wanted to know why. I told her that if she was going to help her daughter, it would be draining on her and she would need a "coach" as well as someone to use for emotional support and guidance. She looked repelled by this last sentence, so I asked her who she did turn to for these conflicts. She explained that at forty years of age, she was fully independent and didn't need anyone to turn to. I responded that we had met several times and nothing dangerous or damaging had occurred, so we should try this for several sessions. Taking this as a challenge, she agreed. On her way out of the room, she turned to me, smiled, and said with the utmost aplomb, "I do feel that I'm being misread by you, but I always keep my appointments."

The next day, Ronnie called for an appointment. I told her that her pattern of disappearing from treatment meant that something was wrong and that I would like her to meet with a woman psychiatrist for awhile and we could evaluate this after a month. She was surprised but agreed to do it.

The psychiatrist I recommended was someone she had met for medication only after my first session with Ronnie. Ronnie had liked her. I received a call from the psychiatrist, who wanted to make sure that Ronnie's request for an appointment was legitimate and had my approval. I explained that it was indeed legitimate and that I believed Ronnie would be untreatable unless her mother's unaddressed neediness was treated so the mother would allow her daughter to get close to someone else without fearing abandonment.

So far the case is still unresolved.

Further Dangers

Infinite pitfalls await the therapist who treats anorexia nervosa. The most common is worry for the medical and physical safety of the patient. This usually boils down to weight loss. This dangerous condition may dazzle the therapist out of the clinical evenness he or she needs to treat the patient successfully. Another pitfall is lying on the part of the patient. Anorexics use numerous deceptions to affect weight gain or disguise weight loss, from drinking large amounts of water before a weigh-in to loading up with a variety of metal weights in the most surprising and undetectable parts of their bodies, along with the usual weighting of pockets.

On the therapist's part, the reaction that can sabotage treatment earliest is impatience with the patient. Weight loss often continues in the initial stages of treatment. Part of this is to test the therapist's reaction. The patient wants to know how disturbing her behavior is to the therapist and to get the therapist enmeshed in the cycle of anger and guilt she created for her parents. The therapist can't afford to be drawn into this, nor can we be totally indifferent about weight and still create an alliance during the early stages of therapy.

Perhaps the most difficult pitfalls to identify are those that involve a threat to existing family relationships between the patient and one or both of her parents. In these cases, the therapist has to be aware of the conscious and unconscious resistance of family members along with the patient to sabotage treatment. If these pitfalls are not identified and addressed, successful treatment cannot be achieved.

In some cases, the patient may show more flexibility in her eating, appear more outgoing with her friends, get along better at home. These behavioral changes can lull a therapist into a false sense of security. While issues of mood and personality, along with social development, are primary and may be underlying and supporting the structure of the illness, low weight must be given up to gain real access to these issues. Often a parent will call me up and happily inform me that their daughter is in a much better frame of mind, a better mood for the last few days. Then I know the patient is high on losing weight. Other times, the opposite occurs. Parents call me because their daughter is tense and snappy. I usually assume this is because she is struggling with the panic of gaining weight.

These changes are both difficult and confusing to parents. As parents, we want to see our children smiling, relaxed, and happy. We don't want to see them tense, snappy, angry, or sulky. It is especially painful for parents when their children's unhappiness is directed against them, implying that they are the cause. When an anorexic is in treatment, parents are not only anxious and angry but confused. "Good is bad and bad is good." It is a terrible choice to have to make, trading a child's smile for weight gain.

When parents and therapists can avoid these and other dangers that prevent recovery, they are also sending a message to their child that they have faith in the child to tolerate the frightening, to face the difficult in order to change her life for the better—to save her life.

CORA AND LENA

Cora was the daughter of a harsh, alcoholic mother called Margo. She was an abused and neglected child. She lived with her sister Laura in a large country house; her mother was married to a wealthy businessman who had an apartment in the city where he claimed he needed to be several days a week to court clients. Margo was alone with the two daughters most of the week. She drank much of the daytime and was usually angry and abusive to the girls for one reason or another. If they came home from school late, they were locked out of the house until they had gathered a sufficient store of kindling wood for the next several days. Margo liked a fire burning in one of their four fireplaces all the time. Often Margo would hit her daughters; once she broke Cora's arm, and another time she broke Laura's nose by flinging her against the refrigerator door. It was nearly a mile from the end of their driveway to where the school bus would pick them up. Often Margo didn't want to bother to drive them even in rain or snow and the girls had to run the distance to catch their school bus.

Cora knew how *not* to raise children. She would never allow her daughters to feel the way she had felt as a child. She had become aware, as an adolescent, that she was raised differently from her friends. As a child, she thought that her mother's demands and punishments were probably the same as other mothers'. When she became part of a peer group as an adolescent, and other kids began to talk about the way they were raised, the complaints they had, Cora realized how much more severely her mother treated her and her sister than other mothers treated their children. She was saddened, since she felt that this meant her mother did not love or value her as much as other mothers valued their children. In addition, her father's frequent absences, and his ignorance or disinterest in the way Margo treated the girls, supported Cora's idea that the girls deserved this treatment. During her childhood she believed this was normal, though she hated it. During adolescence, she became depressed that she was of so little value to her parents that they could treat her this way.

When Cora married, she vowed to herself that if she ever had children, they would feel valued by her and her husband, Harold. Soon, her daughter, Lena, was born and she seemed a happy child, often hugged, kissed, and enjoyed by both parents. Lena was also a nurturing child herself. Even as a three-year-old she would compliment her mother on the way she dressed, how pretty she was, or if Cora looked tired after a day at work. Cora adored Lena, sometimes wishing that her daughter and she were friends instead of mother and daughter. Cora worried most about invitations that would take Lena away from home—whether for the afternoon, day, or later, overnight. In adolescence, Lena seemed to become extremely independent. She sought to participate in events that took her away from home. Cora argued and often forbade her to go. The arguments became more frequent, to the confusion of Harold, who watched the mother-daughter relationship evolve from mutual adoration to a battling mother with a sullen daughter.

Lena developed anorexia at the age of fifteen. She decided that her younger sister was prettier, and this was not acceptable to her. Her sister was taller and thinner, more acceptable in today's culture. Lena began to lose weight—one more issue for Cora and Lena to argue about. Somehow this allowed Lena to argue with her mother without feeling guilty that she was damaging her mother. Previously, all the issues they argued about made Lena guilty as well as angry. This was a particularly attractive issue because Lena could feel assertive without feeling guilty.

After meeting with Cora, and Lena separately, I requested that all three of them come in together. I had not spoken to Harold, Cora's husband, except for a brief telephone conversation.

Lena showed up first, on time. I asked her into the office. She was thin but just about on the borderline between normal and suspicious-looking. At five foot four, she weighed one hundred pounds (I weigh my anorexic patients in the office), down from one hundred and twenty.

"I'm glad they aren't here yet," Lena commented.

"Why is that?"

"I just wanted to clue you in to watch how ready my mother is to spring at me over anything. She gets so angry over anything I say and do, whether it's important or not."

"If I see that I'll bring it right up on the spot," I assured her. "The same way I bring everything up that I observe happening between people here."

"Okay. I've got nothing to hide. I know I'm mad at them because they don't let me do anything my friends do. And I know that she's jealous that I talk to my friend's mother and ask her for advice more than I do my own mother. I just don't trust her anymore."

Just then Cora and Harold arrived. Cora's expression changed from anger to pity and exasperation. Lena forced a smile.

"Did you have a good day at school today, dear?"

"Yeah, it was okay."

I interrupted, "Lena and I were just discussing how members of the family feel when they talk to each other, especially when they argue with each other. Maybe it would be useful for Lena to repeat what she just said to me. Would you do that, Lena?"

Lena, looking a little embarrassed and unprepared for my witnessing what happened between herself and her mother, began haltingly, "Well . . . I was just saying that I never feel just one thing about you. I always feel a bunch of things at once, so I don't know what to say to you or how to say it."

Cora's wounded look was unmistakable. Her eyes became shiny but she did not allow herself to cry. She marshaled her strength and asked Lena, "What are all these different things that you feel at once, Lena?"

"Mostly I feel mad at you and sorry for you," Lena said, looking at the floor.

Cora's tears started to fall. It was too much for her; she had tried too hard as a mother for it to end up like this. But Cora fought her way through the tears and calmly asked her daughter, "Why do you feel sorry for me?"

At that point, Lena started to cry. "I don't know. I get so mad at you for setting too many rules. Sometimes I think that your rules are just to keep me closer to you and prevent me from growing up. I feel like I want to grow up, but if I do, then I'll be doing something terrible to you. So I'm often angry at you and feeling sorry for you, but then I hate myself for the whole thing. I guess I'm the only person in my life that I'm safe to be mad at."

Cora looked shocked. "I've tried so hard not to set harsh rules for you."

"You don't set harsh rules. You're never mean to me. You just set rules that seem to keep me close to you. Rules won't keep us close to each other. I don't know what will, but your rules won't. I want to run away from you and at the same time I'm afraid to leave you. I'm not even sure if I'm afraid to leave you for myself or for you."

At this point there was mutual crying and spontaneous hugging.

The hugging was brief. It ended abruptly, as if Lena had a change of heart, or her feelings of affection evaporated. She moved to the other end of the couch. Cora took it gracefully, as though the exchange had a more natural ending than it did. She wiped her tears and returned to a hint of a smile. Her daughter's face took on a blank expression.

"What just happened?" I inquired.

Lena volunteered, "We had a warm moment together."

I scratched my head and looked puzzled. "It seemed quite momentary from my perspective. Do you have lots of warm moments, and are they all so brief?"

I was looking at Lena. She caught my stare. Her blank expression burst into angry energy, directed to her mother. "You see, that's what I *mean*—about myself, that is! One second I feel mad at you, the next second I feel sorry for you and warm to you, and in another instant I'm repelled by you." Lena looked ashamed that she had used such a harsh word to end her statement, but she remained silent after saying it, indicating that she was not revoking it.

Cora was clearly hurt. She tried to recover by attempting to reassure her daughter that "All teenagers feel that way, dear, don't allow these feelings to make you feel like a bad person."

Lena replied firmly, "All teenagers do *not* feel like that! I'm not even sure it makes me feel like a bad person—sometimes. But what if it's not me? What if it's you? I mean, I think you're weird."

Cora responded, having recovered from her wound, "All I have to say about that is that almost *all* teenagers think their parents are weird, square, out of touch, and a bunch of other things."

"No, I don't mean any of those things. I mean, you are weird with me. I don't care if you're in touch with the latest music. I think you're afraid of me. I think you've always been afraid of something about me. I don't think you can be straight with me about who you are, what you feel, or how you feel about me, ever."

Cora looked stunned. She thought for a minute. The heretofore silent Harold stepped in to rescue his wife from his daughter. "Lena, how could you say that about your mother? She's not afraid of you. She's always completely honest with you, she wouldn't lie to you . . ."

"You don't understand! You never do! You're talking on the surface. I'm not talking about what Mom says. I'm talking about what she *feels*, which you never notice because you're out of it. Either you're too tired from work, cocktails, or wine, or you're lost in the football game on TV."

Lena looked exasperated. I asked Harold, "How would you describe the relationship between your daughter and your wife?"

Harold looked puzzled. "Well, I think that they have a pleasant relationship, with the usual bumps or ups and downs."

"The usual ups and downs!" Lena shouted. "How would you know anything about our relationship? You wouldn't know anything about any relationship! You just want it quiet so you can hear the television. What do you know about me?"

Harold looked taken aback by the comprehensiveness and challenge of her question. He sat there fearful of the audience that was his family. "What kind of a question is that? No one could answer it the way you asked it. I know that *you* are moody, distant, and often sullen. I also know that you can be charming, lovely, and lovable. Sometimes, you are nice to your mother. Sometimes, you snap at her over nothing, often, lately. It's usually connected to food, or weight, or your exercising, though. I think that your relationship with your mother has changed since you developed anorexia. I think it has changed your personality and made you miserable. That's why we're here. You are angry at everybody most of the time and especially at your mother. It might be helpful if you did some of the talking and stopped putting your mother and me on the defensive. How are you going to get over this—whatever-you-call-it—disease if you don't tell us who you are, or who you have become?"

Lena didn't answer her father. Cora broke the silence.

"Hal, I think that maybe you're too hard on Lena. We get along all right."

Harold looked frustrated. "Sometimes it feels like the two of you are locking me out. You both like this relationship you have? Great! Cora, you think that I'm too hard on Lena? I think you have a tendency to be her doormat. I can't believe that's doing her any good."

I intervened. "It seems like each of you is protecting Lena from the other. Has it always been like that?"

Cora responded, "Maybe slightly in the past, but much more so since . . . since she developed this problem."

Lena interrupted, "I don't think there's anything wrong with our family . . . or me."

I responded, "Lena, you wouldn't want anything to change in your family, then?"

"I'd like everyone to be more patient with me and stop bugging me."

"But you just stated that you were angry because your father didn't know much about your relationship with your mother."

Lena shrugged.

"So where does this conversation leave us?" Harold asked.

"It shows us that two parents have become divided by an illness that affects their daughter and her illness needs to keep them divided so that the unhealthy, obsessive, anorexic part of her will not be interfered with. In that way the security her illness offers her won't be disrupted."

Cora was offended. "Why should this dangerous, debilitating behavior offer Lena security? That seems like a contradiction. We are the people in her life that keep her safe and secure, not this starvation and deprivation she is doing. That only threatens her physical and emotional security. She looks terrible and she's irritable, sullen, and depressed."

Lena started to cry.

"But she clings to it, doesn't she?" I pointed out.

Now Cora was tearful. "Yes, but why should she when she should be clinging to us instead?"

Lena's eyes widened with anger. "Yes, you would like me to cling to you, to need you, all the time. But it's you who clings to me, so what do you have to offer me?" She began to cry again. "Never mind. I'm sorry."

Everyone looked confused. I interpreted, "Lena, is this what you meant when you said that you have too many feelings about your mother at one time?"

Blowing her nose hard into a tissue, she nodded vigorously.

Cora looked embarrassed. I prodded her a bit. "What do you think about what Lena said?"

Cora responded haltingly, "I know that I love Lena. I am aware of how important she is to me. I never thought of myself as clinging to her or needy for her attention, but she may be right."

"Did *your* mother need you, Cora?" I asked softly.

Cora began to cry. She did so for awhile without talking. We all waited for her to speak.

"I don't think my mother ever needed me for anything but service. From collecting firewood to cleaning the house. She never said thank you. *Never.* Everything was expected of me, nothing was appreciated. I never mattered, except for what I could *not* do correctly. Oh, there was plenty of criticism. There just wasn't any praise. And I'm doing the opposite with Lena. She gets more praise in a day than I got in my whole childhood and adolescence! I seem to get that combination that Lena was talking about. Part of her is nice to me—that part is no doubt what I wished my mother would give me. The other part of her is mean to me, just like my mother was. Can you beat that? I make sure that with my daughter, I do everything the opposite way from my mother, and my daughter gives me the same abuse—well, maybe not quite the same, but the same tone my mother used with me. I feel like an idiot."

Cora's tone had shifted during her response from sad and tearful to straightforwardly angry.

"How does your mother's anger make you feel, Lena?"

Lena was surprised at my shift toward her.

"I don't know. I feel bad in one way because I don't want her to be unhappy, but she sounds strong and unhappy and I like that better than weak and unhappy . . . maybe I'm crazy. I just don't want to be the cause of her unhappiness. I don't want to be responsible for anyone else." She began to cry again. "I can't even take care of myself. Don't they know that?" She wept intensely for a few minutes.

"Cora and Harold, what does it feel like to be told that by your daughter?"

Harold began, "I feel like no one listens to me when I want us, Cora and myself, to take charge of Lena. Now Lena is upset because we haven't. What do you think, honey?"

Cora responded, "I guess maybe you're not so dangerous, Hal. Maybe I'm afraid that you'll become my mother with Lena." She smiled ironically. "It seems that all I've succeeded in doing is getting Lena to act like my mother, sometimes. So how do we break such old habits that we've practiced without knowing it?"

Everyone was looking at me. "I guess by practicing new habits and identifying those old ones every time they pop out of anyone's mouth. It's a lot of work and takes a long time, and worst of all the old habits are more natural, more comfortable for each of you to follow. Hal, it's easy for you to butt out and resent it at the same time. Cora, it's natural for you to want to make it up to the wrong child. You can't make up to Lena what your mother did to you, or didn't do for you. Lena never had your mother to begin with and she can't give you what your mother didn't.

"Now, Lena," I turned to her, "you have a difficult job in changing because of the three of you, you have the most to lose with a change in the family system." Lena looked suspiciously at me. "You have *power* to lose. You have succeeded in 'dividing and conquering' your parents. Your best emotional interest lies in losing power, but nobody wants to voluntarily give up power. The good thing about giving up power is that you gain protection from the people you give it up to . . . if they love you. Do you think that your parents love you?"

Lena reacquired her suspicious look. "Are you trying to trap me?"

"No, we will be taking power away from you whether you like it or not and exchanging it for the emotional protection that you've always secretly wanted."

This case illustrates how a mother can nurture to compensate for her own neediness, while the child can perceive the unconsciously hidden neediness, deny her own needs for self-expression and food, and resentfully punish her mother for sending her a mixed message.

Mothers are not the only targets of an anorexic's rage and disappointment. The next case gives us insight into the (initially) unconscious rage a daughter has toward her father for demeaning her mother, even though he was always distantly pleasant toward the daughter.

SONDRA

Sondra was born in a wealthy suburb of a South American country. Karen, her mother, was the daughter of concentration camp survivors who immigrated to South America before the United States was willing to accept Jews and turned them away. Her father, Eric, was a German Jew whose family fled Germany as soon as Hitler came to power but before the persecution of Jews was official policy. Eric told me proudly that his father had read *Mein Kampf*, saw the handwriting on the wall, packed up his family, and left for the western hemisphere to any country that would take them.

Both Karen's and Eric's parents married in 1946, a year after World War II ended. Karen and Eric were each both born a year later, in 1947. They met and married at the age of twenty, in 1967. They had three children; two sons, Avie and Yakov, and a daughter, Sondra. They would not give the children German names, but by the time Sondra came along they were sufficiently at peace with their new country to give her a Spanish name. Eric was proud like his father and joined a successful international exporting firm.

Karen's father had been a successful, well-paid lawyer in Germany with Daimler-Benz. The combination of his persecution, degradation, and escape to the West, only to find German-speaking lawyers could not get work in a Spanish-speaking country, threw him into a depression that lasted for four years. He gradually worked his way up in the same company that Eric's father worked in. Eric's father held the senior position of the two, but the men were friendly, and when their children met it was instant romance.

Karen always felt that she had married "up"—after all, Eric's father held a superior position in the community as well as the firm, and her own father was always regarded by the family as fragile, though he had recovered from his depression before Karen was born. She always behaved deferentially toward her husband, who in the eyes of their daughter, Sondra, seemed subservient. Sondra also felt he enjoyed his position as patriarch of the family. They moved around, lived in several countries in Europe. Each time they moved, Karen dropped whatever budding business she was developing to accommodate her husband's transfer. Sondra always saw this as a second-class position for her mother. She felt that her father dismissed her work as women's hobbies. Her two brothers did well in school, as did she, proving that everything her father did was correct, especially to her mother.

The family ended up in New Jersey, far from the firm's headquarters, and her father was becoming bitter at what looked like his "dead-end" position in the company. As his confidence declined, he became more critical of his wife. According to Sondra, their relationship deteriorated into her father hurling insults at her mother and her mother's passive acceptance of this.

At the age of fourteen, Sondra developed anorexia nervosa. She was five foot eight and her weight plummeted from a slender one hundred and thirty pounds to a skeletal eighty pounds. During the entire weight-losing period, Sondra cheerfully declared that she didn't care about losing weight and, indeed, never weighed herself. Whatever foods she ate, she ate in front of her family, so that even they were puzzled and panicked by this weight loss. Many physicians were consulted before Sondra was referred to me since she just didn't sound like the other anorexics they had met; she denied wanting to lose weight, stated that she didn't care if she gained weight, was always engaging, smiling, friendly, and seemed just as curious about her weight loss as they were. Finally, finding nothing physically wrong with her, the last physician, who had been her mother's pediatrician in South America, referred her to me as an "atypical anorexic."

Sondra entered the office with an appearance that shocked me. Her limbs were sticklike. Her tendons and veins were visible. Miraculously, her face still looked normal, even pretty. This last detail is what probably delayed the diagnosis. More physicians and parents look at the face to make a health judgment about anorexia than many people realize.

"I understand that you've been seen by many doctors," I began. "You must be a bit weary of all the examinations."

"Yes." She giggled. "I guess they've finally made up their minds about me."

"What do you think about the diagnosis of anorexia nervosa?"

Sondra shrugged. "I guess that's what they think."

"What do *you* think?"

"I don't know. I don't even know how I lost the weight. I wasn't trying to."

"You lost fifty pounds without trying to, or noticing?" I looked amused since I was sure those before me had probably looked infuriated.

"Yes," she replied. "I still don't know how it happened."

I considered two possibilities: first, that she was using denial; second, that she was being extremely guarded on a conscious level. I decided to go with the second. My task would be to help her drop her guard with me or there would be no real therapy happening. If she took all this trouble to deny her deliberate weight loss, then she had no tolerance for straightforward disagreements. There was an angry, upset girl hiding behind the seemingly impregnable smile and giggle.

I asked her, "Do you get angry with members of your family and tell them that you're angry?"

"It depends on what it's about."

"What are the safer things to argue?"

"Oh, if someone is late, or borrows something of mine without asking. Stuff like that."

"What would be a really difficult subject to express your anger about?"

She paused, glanced at the ceiling, then looked me in the eye, shrugged, and said, "I don't really know. I never thought about it."

"Are there aspects of relationships—how people get along within the family—that bother you?"

"Well, no family is perfect. I suppose there must be some things that bother me."

"Can you think of anything specific?"

She looked exaggeratedly puzzled, cocking her head to one side, furrowing her eyebrows, bringing her upper lip down at the corners; quite a display.

"I can't think of anything right now. I'm sure I'll think of something later, though."

Her avoidance was exquisite. She pleasantly discouraged confrontation.

"Who do you cry to?"

She seemed surprised by the question.

"My mother, I guess."

"Who do you cry to about yourself, your disappointments about the way your life is working out?"

"My life is working out fine. What do you mean?"

"You are fourteen years old, embattled with your parents and doctors about your eating and weight. Your appearance suggests that you are eating one-half to one-third of what your body needs. Did you ever imagine that this would dominate your life, say, two years ago?"

She shook her head sadly.

"So, when you are saying to me, cheerfully, that everything is all right, you are ignoring all the things in your life and family that are going wrong. Why do you need to do that?"

"Well, I don't know you very well."

"When you are with your brothers, or your parents, who you *do* know very well, do you discuss thoughts and feelings that you have about yourself?"

"I don't know what there is to discuss with them."

"So, we have a deeper problem. You have no thoughts to realize your feelings. That means you have to act them out numbly like cheerfully losing weight to a near-death situation without thinking about the anger toward those who want you to stop, or fearing the dangerous condition of your health."

"I guess so," she nodded, conceding the point.

This was unusual. I was treating someone who wasn't just resistant but had no language to articulate her own feelings, or her own anger. In addition, she was guarded about the possibility that she could harbor unacceptable thoughts against herself, as well as others. I would have to teach Sondra a language that she could use to express her feelings and hope I was correct.

But first I would have to convince her to develop a sense that this was necessary and that something was actually wrong. I made her stand in front of a full-length mirror. She was wearing shorts and a sleeveless top. I tilted the mirror so she could not see her head or face.

"If you saw another girl who looked like this, what would you think of her appearance?"

She stared in silence for a moment, looking the figure up and down, stopping briefly at shoulders, thighs, and calves. Finally she looked at me. "She's very thin."

"Too thin?" I inquired. "Would you want your mother to look like that?"

A tear trickled down her right cheek. "No, I guess not."

"Do *you* find this appearance acceptable to yourself?"

"Maybe I have smaller bones," she responded dispassionately.

"Is it important that no one knows how you feel?"

"Maybe."

I smiled. "The perfect yes."

"What do you mean?"

"I asked you if you needed to conceal your communications about feelings and you concealed the answer to my question."

"Oh," she said flatly.

"Do *you* know how you feel?"

"About what?"

"Yourself, your parents, your brothers?"

"I love them."

"Is that the extent of your awareness of your feelings toward your family?"

"Yes. Everything is all right."

"What do you think about during the course of the day?"

"What I have to do that day."

"What do you think about on weekends or vacations?"

"Nothing."

"What did you think about yesterday?"

"Nothing."

"What were you thinking about before our session today, or even earlier today?"

"Nothing."

"What kind of mood or moods were you in today?"

"Okay, the usual."

I did not feel Sondra was trying to conceal anything from me, but I did believe it was intensely important that she conceal the answers to my questions, or even the idea of such questions from *herself*.

During the first year of therapy, she gave many "Yes," "No," and "Okay" answers. I responded with explanations about how other girls might answer the questions to build in a frame of reference to allow these ideas to become acceptable, even thinkable.

Occasionally, when I felt that the answer to a question would not pose conflict, I would inquire if a hypothetical answer I provided might apply to her. To my surprise, she would give me a definite "Yes." Her "Yes" became more frequent. I call this stage "chiming in." For example, "Do you feel uninteresting?"

"Yes."

Now it would be time to encourage Sondra to initiate responses without me being the questioner and answerer. A very small portion of each session was devoted to eating and weight. I had to explain to Sondra how her talk changed her and fostered growth. During this first year, she had gained twenty pounds.

She questioned me about this idea of her talking being so important.

"I like it when you explain what I don't understand about myself. I'm amazed how you can tell me what bothers me. But if I don't know what it is, why can't I depend on you for that information? And besides, I'm embarrassed to say this, but when you talk to me about myself, it reminds me of the time my mother used to read bedtime stories to me. It feels good."

"I talk to you about yourself so that you build a storehouse of conscious ideas and words that you didn't have before. This collection of ideas you have will give you a reference point to make your own statements about yourself. When you talk to me, there are two listeners, you and me. Your talk becomes a declaration, a fact. When you hear yourself, what you say becomes more real than when you only think it silently. You feel the truth of what you have said. It follows that you feel a little differently about yourself. All these little differences add up over time. The result is that you trust yourself, you feel more real to yourself, you believe in yourself, and you are less afraid of yourself—even parts of yourself that you don't yet understand."

"Does that mean you will stop talking to me when we meet?"

"No, it means that I will ask you to do more of the initiating talk and I will do less. The 'bad' news is that now I have more faith in you to do this, so I will push you harder to talk, and I'll probably tease you about being guarded when you don't answer."

"Oh great, now this all gets worse for me."

"No, now you start to grow at a faster rate."

"What if you're wrong and I can't do what you expect?"

"Then we will back up to a point where you can do what I expect. You're so used to seeing everything as all or nothing."

As time went on, Sondra and I would talk about the feelings that created the climate for developing anorexia. Considering where we started, the complexity of her interpretations surprised me.

"My father always had a big important corporate job which just continued to get bigger and more important as he got promoted. Every time he got a promotion we moved—six times. Six times I had to make new friends. I guess that kept my brothers and me closer. My mother would set up businesses wherever he was transferred to. When she protested that another transfer would eradicate all her efforts in her new business, he would make fun of her, devalue her business and her intelligence. He was always so superior and smug. It was as if he tried to make her feel stupid. I think that he liked believing he was the only one who could do things right and *everything* he did was perfect. Well, I wasn't going to be perfect. My thinness was proof that he couldn't be such a great father and still have such a skinny, ugly daughter."

"Then your anorexia was your getting revenge for your mother against the way your father treated her?"

"Yes, I guess it was—and still is. That's why I don't gain the rest of the weight, so he can't feel so good about himself."

"But you've said that a lot of that has changed and at this point in his career he turns to her for advice and treats her with respect almost always."

"Yes, that's true, but I'm very sensitive to any time he doesn't; maybe I'm oversensitive. It seems like they've gotten better and I'm still stuck. It's unfair."

"What about her?"

"What do you mean?"

"If he can't feel like an adequate father because of your illness, how can she feel the self-esteem a successful mother feels? It seems despite what she got back from his changed behavior and their changed relationship, your illness keeps her bound closer to you in a worried and needy way."

"You mean I'm doing the same kind of damage to her that he used to?"

"Kind of."

"Oh, this is terrible! Then I really do have to gain the rest of the weight back! How do I do it?"

"You have to eat into the storm of anxiety you feel when you know you have eaten more than it takes to maintain your present weight. If you don't feel guilty about eating too much, then you haven't eaten enough. I have to weigh you every week to see if you have tolerated enough anxiety."

"That's the worst offer anyone's ever made me."

"I'm sure it is. But I think that I'm supposed to make you this offer and you're supposed to take me up on it."

"When I've gained the weight, then what? Then who will I be?"

"An adolescent student catching up with all you missed out on during the three years you had this illness, and I'll help you catch up."

"You better."

The next stage of treatment involved two aspects: to coax Sondra's weight up to one hundred and ten pounds—ten more pounds than she currently weighed and twenty less than her pre-anorexic weight. And to work with her parents.

The work with her parents was done by another therapist—mostly with her mother, which strengthened her position in the relationship with the father. Now the mother would have to show that she was not so needy that she had to telephone her daughter three times a day at college, and discontinue other behaviors that would keep mother and daughter clinging to each other.

Every child begins life with the legacy of a gene pool that is the synthesis of its ancestors, going back to the beginning of the human species. At the same time, every child is born with a potentially clean slate of human experiences. That child may have projected upon it the identities of others in its parents' lives: people who affected its parents. Parents need to parent that child with no unconscious fears, no leftover grudges from other relationships, no extreme reactions to compensate for the parents' own childhood. Each child deserves love, reasonableness, structure, limits, protection, and warmth, all in some healthy balance. The closer parents come to this nearly unattainable ideal, the healthier the way that the child with the clean slate can develop.

We all read and talk about working through marital relationships as a lifetime job. We will also have to add that working through parent-child relationships is a lifetime job, too.

14

HOSPITALIZATION

A GOOD friend, and a distinguished psychiatrist, commented to me one day, "You know, I had the strangest experience today. A friend of mine was placed in the psychiatric unit of my hospital. It's a unit where I've treated inpatients for over fifteen years. Whenever I walk in, the door locks behind me, somewhat noisily, but I pay no attention to it. Today, I went to the unit during visiting hours—as a visitor this time, to see my friend. When the door lock clicked behind me, I felt locked in, I became anxious and began to perspire—in my own unit! I was a civilian for the moment, and it didn't feel good."

We do not enter hospitals casually. If we have to go to an acute care medical hospital where diagnoses are made, surgery done, and medical emergencies treated, along with chronic and fatal diseases, we usually experience tension. If we are lucky enough not to be the patient admitted, our tension increases with the importance of the patient to us, and the seriousness of his or her condition.

In 1974, I was invited by a teaching hospital to treat patients hospitalized with anorexia nervosa. I had no medical training and felt very much a "civilian" in an intimidating setting. It was a time when there were no eating disorder programs and no place had much institutional experience in treating them. The nurses were annoyed with the "neurotic brats that wouldn't eat" while other patients were in pain, bleeding, or terminal. At that time, the staff's task was to keep the anorexic from dying, put some weight on them, and send them home—"Good riddance!" The medical students made their daily rounds continually asking these girls questions to determine their sanity (Mental Status Evaluation), and other questions about why they didn't want to eat. It was the job of each medical student to do the routine for his or her medical education, not to treat the patient.

No one knew what treatment was appropriate. If the patient was dangerously thin, she was bullied into eating, put on a nasogastric tube, or fed through her jugular vein, through a catheter that was stitched onto the skin above it and bandaged to avoid infection (hyperalimentation). These, of course, are emergency measures, and back in the seventies we had nothing but emergencies. No one recognized anorexia nervosa until a girl was dangerously emaciated. Up to that point she just looked a bit skinnier than the fashion models of the times. Very few people, including psychiatrists or medical professionals, had seen or heard about anorexia nervosa.

I asked the doctor who invited me to work with the anorexic patients why he had selected me, a nonmedical person. His answer was simple. "We've got a federal grant and you've got the patients."

The first patient I ever requested to be hospitalized (with her pediatrician's encouragement) begged me not to put her in the hospital. As a therapist, no one ever "begged" me for anything before. She cried and promised that she would eat more and gain weight if only I wouldn't "put her in there." Using power did not sit well with me. I offered her one last chance, which would last a week, to gain weight and avoid hospitalization. She assured me she would—and didn't. I had to call her mother and tell her that her daughter needed hospitalization. The girl cried while I made the call, in her presence.

I was supposed to be demanding, or commanding, or whatever. Instead, I felt frightened, bad, guilty, and a failure. I did manage to cling to a sensible ethic for this strategy, which I had to repeat many times during her tear-filled session. "You are in danger, whether you believe it or not, of dying. Dr. — — — has verified this and we have to stop you from dying. It is obvious that you can't stop yourself, and I can't stop you in an outpatient setting. So you must go into the hospital."

I called the hospital, after speaking with her mother, and they asked me what were to become the usual admission questions for me. "What is the patient's name, address, date of birth, Social Security number, health insurance company, policy number," and so on.

It was an odd experience. I was instructing her to go to a hospital that might save her life without curing her. Like most laypeople in 1974, I assumed that hospitals "cured" patients—sent them home fixed, repaired permanently. I was about to be co-opted into a system I was unprepared for, but not as unprepared as the hospitals were to receive my patients. Back in what I will have to refer to as the "good old days," a patient could be kept in a hospital until doctors felt she was ready to leave without relapsing. This usually took three months or more. Today, three weeks is the time limit for hospital stay.

Gradually, the earlier diagnosis of anorexia in individuals reduced the need for medical interventions I have described in which twenty-four-hour, seven-day-a-week care and supervision were necessary. This care shifted to the psychiatric hospitals. Eating disorder programs were developed and improved upon through the eighties. Today's increasing limitations on inpatient stay, and lower staff-to-patient ratios, have reduced the likelihood of success and lowered staff morale. This makes the quality of improvement for the patient lower and poorer.

Most institutions designated "hospitals" or "psychiatric hospitals" have similar protocols: They have to treat the patient behaviorally, observing and reporting her eating intake and granting privileges dependent on weight gain. The privileges may range from being allowed to leave one's room to not having to wear bed clothes to eating real food instead of liquid diets. Failure to comply with the weight gain often invites the punishment of nasogastric feeding, which simply put means a tube is inserted into the patient's nose and as much as five hundred calories of liquid diet is "poured" into that tube, which ends up in her stomach or duodenum. Then she is watched for over an hour to make sure that she doesn't throw up the food. While in the hospital, this protocol is nearly 100 percent successful. After discharge, however, the statistics change. Hospitals also have exploratory family therapy sessions, and multiple family groups, which invite parents and siblings to explore their own feelings about having an anorexic child or sibling.

A well-coordinated psychiatric program gives the anorexic patient and her family a "leg up," a boost in the direction of recovery. Psychiatric hospitalization offers several other advantages to the downward-spiraling anorexic. Thorough diagnostic work can be done to see if the patient has other psychiatric disorders which may need to be treated as well. These may range from anxiety, depression, manic-depression, and borderline personality disorder, to thought disorder (schizo-phreniform categories), and others, all of which will be more apparent in an environment where someone can be observed continuously. Hospitals, because of their authoritarian structure, can discreetly medicate and evaluate the effectiveness of the medication more quickly than an outpatient setting. Hospitalization also provides often-needed separation of patient from family so both can reorganize for change.

I am of course talking about a well-organized and well-run hospital when I describe these conditions and advantages even for short-term hospitalization. Even so, events are imperfect and treatment will benefit some patients more than others. Often, the youngest patients in a unit benefit the least if there is a wide age range. They may be more influenced by the pathology of the older patients than by the staff. Most hospitals gear their general rules and procedures to deal with the most symptomatic and most disturbed patients. Frequently, it is these patients who will show the most improvement. This does not mean they will leave the hospital in optimum health; that would be unrealistic.

When considering any short-term psychiatric treatment, it is important to remember that it has taken many years for someone to develop his or her personality and a larger portion of that time to form the foundation for mental illness than would seem apparent. A major consideration in looking at the entire treatment picture, if hospitalization is part of that picture, is what treatment following discharge will be necessary to continue satisfactory progress toward recovery. Should the patient be transferred to a day program, which will have many of the components of the hospital program but with the patient going home at the end of the day and returning the next morning, on a five-day-a-week basis? Should the patient join a support group (discussed in chapter 16)? In all cases, intensive individual psychotherapy will be necessary to help the patient adjust to the changes she has gone through in the hospital; to continue to work on her deficits in the areas of trust, dependency, and attachment; and to continue to develop an awareness about her identity, femininity, and intimacy, among other problems.

Looking back over the past twenty-five years, I have seen encouraging changes from the time when there was no field of eating disorders to the present, when we have networks of professionals and several professional journals, as well as volunteer agencies for referral sources (see Appendix B) and a popular awareness that makes early identification prevalent, and acceptable.

Twenty-nine years ago, I saw my first anorexic. Twenty-four years ago, I treated my first hospitalized patient. Those first few years were trying for everyone involved in treatment.

NORA

At my first teaching hospital, I was treating two patients when I noticed an emaciated, slattern-faced fifteen-year-old stalking me in the corridors of the hospital. She kept her distance but was reliably nearby. One day the chairman of the department called me in and said, "Steve, Nora has been on this floor for eighteen months. She has anorexia. She's five feet tall, weighs fifty-five pounds, and is the best manipulator of staff we have ever encountered. She can talk a staff member out of taking blood. She's so savvy about the procedures here that she argues medicine with our interns and residents—and wins. The result is, she gains no weight, the staff is discouraged, and since the family has no money and no insurance, it's taking a huge chunk out of our departmental budget. I'm asking you to treat her as a favor to the department."

Now I had to pursue my stalker and invite her into treatment. Nora, as well as the rest of her family, had a poor personal history. We knew her parents had an unhappy marriage; her mother had attempted suicide by jumping in front of a train and was now confined to a wheelchair. Her father rarely visited. The family seemed to take Nora's hospitalization for granted and to have given up hope that she would ever get well.

Nora was a tough, street-smart kid. She had been to eleven therapists. I would be the twelfth. The most encouraging sign was her interest in me, manifested by her following me and ducking behind doorways when I checked to see if she was still there. One day I switched roles with her and the hunted became the hunter. I spotted her ducking into a patient's room while following me. I did an about-face and walked into the room. I looked at the patient, greeted her (most of the patients on the floor recognized me), and then turned to Nora, who was staring at the patient, avoiding my eyes.

"You're Nora, aren't you?" Now she stared at the floor but did not respond to my question. "I notice that you like to walk up and down the corridors a lot to burn calories. Why don't I join you for awhile? We could talk and I could use the exercise."

She tensed at my reference to her motive. I continued, "I mostly use the stairs instead of these elevators. They take forever to arrive and the ride is boring. Do you take the stairs?" My question was casual. She knew it was a trap, but after being totally secretive to every adult in her life for the past eighteen months, she was bursting to tell someone something about herself.

"I can't use the stairs when I'm on an IV." She indicated with her index finger the metal pole that stood a bit taller than her, with the glucose bottle and tube ending at the needle inserted into her wrist. There seemed like an excessive amount of tape to hold it in place. She noticed my surprise at the amount of tape and smiled shyly. "I guess they don't trust me with IVs. They think I'll pull them out." I nodded, with my best mischievous smile, peering over the top of my glasses. "And do you?" She shrugged her shoulders.

She had told me a lot for a first session: her walking, her use of the stairs—a clear rule-breaker—and finally her pulling out IVs. I didn't want to push her into retreat. She had to regain the feeling that she was the pursuer and not the pursued. I walked a little faster than she could with her IV pole and slowed down for her to catch up every thirty seconds. When I thought she had said enough, I turned to her and said, "I'll be here on Thursday, catch you then." It was still too early to make her an "official" patient. I was number twelve and wanted to be the last therapist.

By our third meeting, Nora was official. We had made an appointment, and we weren't walking in the hallway but instead sat in my office talking. By our sixth meeting, it was time for Nora to test me and deal with her fear of attachment.

I was standing at the nurses' station, writing chart notes, when the senior floor nurse, a strict woman with an Eastern European accent, walked up to me hurriedly, tapped me on the shoulder, and said, "I think you better see this." She indicated with her head and hand in the same direction, Nora's room.

I walked in to see Nora sitting on her bed, a broken IV bottle near her feet. The tubing leading from her wrist was red its full length, and there was a puddle of blood amid the broken glass that had contained the IV fluid. A nurse's aide was cleaning up fluid, blood, and glass. The tubing had been clamped to prevent the continual outflow of blood.

The strict nurse stood there, pointing her index finger at Nora and shouting that this was no accident. The patient didn't even call a staff member when it happened. It was the sound of breaking glass that caught a medical student's attention. She could have bled to death in a few minutes, this "Skinny-malink." I looked at Nora, smiled, and said casually, "So now you know the tube flows both ways." I nodded to her as if she had made a positive discovery and walked out.

I had to arrange two meetings. The first with my chairman, the second with the house staff: medical students, interns, and residents. The institution part of the treatment program would have to begin and I was ready for it.

I walked into my chairman's office. The respect he had earned from his staff made him close to a deity. One could pose him a five-minute summary of a problem and he would respond with a concise sentence that answered every issue raised. I had to ask his permission to threaten to restrain a patient on a nonpsychiatric floor. He looked up at me from his desk, stacked with papers. "Mike," I tried to sound assertive, "Nora is impossible to treat in a setting where she is the most powerful person. I am confining her to her bed for a week except for trips to the bathroom. If she violates those rules, I want her restrained, hands and feet, to the bed. I want to tell her that."

Mike put his head in his hands. I felt like I was asking the impossible, which made me a pain in the neck to him. Then he looked up at me and said, "I don't think that I can do that on a nonpsych unit, but you can threaten her with it, and if she breaks the rules, we'll have her certified and transfer her to the psych unit where they *can* do that. We'll give them medical support so she won't be in danger, and she'll lose you as her therapist, probably the greatest punishment of all. Go threaten her. I'll explain it to the staff." He always knew the answers.

Nora looked at me from her bed, asking incredulously, "If I leave my bed, you'll have me tied to it?"

I looked back at her coolly. "Wrists and ankles."

"Boy, you're tough." She didn't seem displeased with my draconian threat of punishment.

I added, "Every morning at eight-thirty blood will be drawn and you are not to tell the technician or medical student that it's unnecessary, or that it's already been done. It gets done every morning, without fail. Your vital signs will be checked as well. All urine goes into that jug." I indicated with my left hand the gallon jug by the side of her bed. She looked at the narrow neck of the jug and protested, "I can't pee into that. It'll go all over the floor."

"We'll get you one you *can* pee into and pour that into the jug. I'll see you Thursday. I hope I don't hear about you before then." I walked out, having just behaved in the most dictatorial and intrusive manner in my life. None of my training had prepared me for this, but Nora would be lost if I didn't act at least as tough and independent as she was.

My next meeting was with the house staff. This meeting was attended by the chairman as well as those on the floor, along with the students, interns, and residents.

I looked at all these young faces. Suddenly the doctors felt like the junior counselors in a summer camp and I was the head counselor. I felt old. "There is a fifteen-year-old girl who's been on this floor for a year and a half." Everyone knew who I meant. "She still weighs fifty-five pounds. This means that she eats very little food so she must have eaten eighteen rotations of house staffs instead, during the past year and a half." Everyone laughed nervously. "There is no appropriate treatment setting for her. Psych is not prepared for her particular medical emergency, and we are not staffed here for the kind of psych supervision she needs. But we're going to do it here. These will be the rules:

"No one may address a request by her to leave her bed except to use the bathroom.

"She will be observed in the bathroom by a female staff member to make sure she is not vomiting, doesn't have diarrhea, and isn't monkeying with her intravenous line.

"No one will accept any medical information about this patient from herself. No self-reporting unless it is collaborated at the nurses' desk.

"No one will accept her quoting another staff member's comments or orders unless it is verified by the nurses' desk or her chart. She lies. It's part of her disease.

"Your response to any question from her is, 'I'll check with nursing.'

"Her meals will be observed by a dietitian, who will record all liquids and solids she eats.

"Twenty-four-hour urine samples will be collected every day to make sure she's not vomiting despite our precautions.

"While we can't really do it, we must give her the impression that everything she does is observed. That feeling will be her protection from all the impulses this disease plagues her with."

A chain is only as strong as its weakest link. On a pediatric/adolescent medicine floor in 1974, no doctors wanted to police their patients. They became pediatricians because they liked children.

By the third day of this protocol, Nora had been completely cooperative. She even seemed calmer to staff. Her private physician was visiting her when she charmingly asked, "Why am I being treated this way?" He slipped a bit and in a slightly high-pitched voice answered defensively "Steve thinks this is best."

She told me about it the next day, imitating his voice. She didn't want any chinks in the staff's armor, either. Staying with my own protocol, I asked him if her story was true. He nodded and smiled meekly. I always thought he was the toughest doctor on the floor.

Nora continued to behave according to the rules and began to gain weight. In three months, she had gained nearly thirty pounds and was discharged to my outpatient care. She saw me for two years and then left the area. To my knowledge, she never relapsed.

That's where we were in 1974.

During the 1980s the public became more aware, fostering earlier identification. The psychiatric establishment became familiar with both psychological and medical aspects of the disease and "eating disorders units" sprang up throughout the country, each with a different emphasis, each often suitable for patients presenting differing degrees of difficulty, ability to cooperate, additional psychiatric complications, and differing levels of medical endangerment. During this period, hospitals were given the time they needed (by insurance companies) to form staff alliances with patients, no easy task, and then within these treatment alliances, to coerce patients into giving up their self-destructive weight-losing behaviors.

By 1990, the effects of the Wall Street crash of 1987 had reverberated to the health care sector, striking psychiatric hospitals first since they were the most expensive unit on the benefits list. Eating disorders were redlined first. They were considered chronic, and medical economics dictated that allowed hospital stays be reduced if the patient was no longer medically endangered. This step makes relapse likely even with the best-trained and best-intentioned staffs.

Still, minimal as the time allotment is, the patient can benefit from a short encounter with a well-trained staff who can create the therapeutic paradox: a treatment alliance with a patient that they will have to coerce, in a short-term hospitalization.

This might give the patient that start she needs to create momentum and to give her family and the outpatient therapist an opportunity to build on this "leg up" to continue her progress.

However, if today's hospital stays were not just brief episodes of treatment, longer stays in fact might prove less costly, to prevent relapses in many cases, which require rehospitalization.

In the 1980s, many hospitals were approaching optimal treatment models that allowed enough time for the anorexic patient to make an adequate start on the road to recovery.

These components consist of:

—A period of one to two weeks for the patient to become used to hospital routine.

—A far different environment from her home. These differences include supervision; enforceable rules (instead of impotent threats); group living, lack of privacy, even in the bathroom; limitation of possessions, such as sharp objects, blade razors, etc.; and most important of all, the absence of parents.

—Individual psychotherapy (usually three times a week). The sessions are used to create an alliance between the patient and the hospital unit's system of procedures and rules, also to create a relationship in which the patient can (though limited compared to outpatient therapy) rely on the therapist for questions she has about her feelings being a patient subject to hospital routines, and especially about eating and gaining weight. She may also want to talk to her individual therapist about issues relating to her parents, siblings, friends, and school relationships. Often, limitations on time prevent more analytical explorations of how she sees her development in terms of trust, dependency, identity, and femininity.

—Family therapy sessions held once a week when possible, including both parents (if this is feasible), and siblings. Here issues of all pairs of relations (dyads) are discussed as well as the general "mood" of the house.

—Multiple family groups, where all the families in treatment share their problems and issues, as well as the ways they handle them, along with the changes they are experiencing.

—Group therapy, where only those suffering from anorexia nervosa are invited (although sometimes bulimics are included). We have found that when groups include members with other problems but do not include eating disorders, all eating disorder discussion disappears.

—Supervised eating, which means a staff member monitors the food intake, meal by meal, of each patient. This is usually done in a group eating situation in either the unit dining area or the general dining room where eating-disordered patients sit at their own designated tables.

— A privilege system based on weight gain and general cooperation. This is defined by a status given each patient which determines trips outside their unit or the hospital, how much privacy they are allowed, etc.

— Staff conferences, in which every member of the unit staff involved in supervising the patient sits down together several times a week (depending upon the particular hospital) so that the patient's progress and/or difficulties may be evaluated. The staff group also evaluates the patient's efforts to "split" staff members as she did at home, playing Mommy off against Daddy. Other accompanying disorders, where they exist, are evaluated: general anxiety disorders, psychotic episodes, schizophrenia, bipolar illness, obsessive-compulsive disorder, and so on. Treatments, especially medications, are discussed as assisting recovery.

— Recreational activities, physical therapy, and educational coordination with the patient's school (if appropriate)

— Medical monitoring of the patient's weight, vital signs, organ functions, especially kidney and bowel, along with heart and liver, to help the staff evaluate safety and progress, since tampering with health via vomiting, laxatives, or diuretics will be detected.

— Community meetings with the general patient population to foster integration with people not suffering from an eating disorder; this is a first step toward reintegrating with the rest of society after discharge from the hospital.

— Discharge planning, which includes: planned daily activities that may range from day hospital to group meetings to individual psychotherapy at least once a week. When medication is involved, medication follow-up is essential. Educational or employment follow-up, family relationship evaluation, and of course weight and medical follow-ups are all imperative. Discharge from the hospital then is merely what we call a "step down" in treatment, which continues for an indefinite period of time. If all emotional issues are followed up on and dealt with, the likelihood of relapse drops from a national average of 75 percent to less than 10 percent.

This is a complicated process, involving professionals, patients, and family, and demanding time and energy from all. It is no wonder insurance companies run from the prospect of this kind of hospitalization, which is out of the financial reach of most families.

Such an intense hospitalization program may seem harsh, but it treats the core of anorexia for the duration of inpatient treatment, that core being isolation/obsessionality. So much external authority, interference, and direction is provided that the patient's obsessional habits are drowned out. Relinquishing them puts the patient more at east about changing eating patterns and gaining weight than she could accomplish on her own. All this positive interference pays off in the end. Again, I should stress that it is grounded in a well-trained staff and competent unit that has a professional and positive attitude toward their role in the patient's recovery.

15

PREGNANCY

AND THE

RECOVERED ANOREXIC

Facing Pregnancy

HAVE been asked by many anxious parents of teenagers with anorexia, "Will she ever be able to have children?" We have lots of endocrinological research (Catherine Halmi, et al., New York Hospital White Plains) that reproductive hormones can return to normal levels after anorexia. If the patient has not skipped her menstrual periods for more than three years, she will probably be capable of pregnancy and childbirth—when she is ready.

I have been fortunate in that girls I have treated in their teens and early twenties, after they have married and become pregnant, contacted me and requested prenatal psychotherapy (and sometimes postnatal as well). This is often eight to ten years later. Typically, they will come in, sit down, and say to me, "I don't have to be skinny anymore but I'm afraid of my reaction to this," pointing to their abdomens, and drawing a profile arc in the air with their index finger indicating the size they anticipate reaching in a few months.

This poses a marvelous opportunity to view both the afteraffects of anorexia on motherhood, and the "birth of motherhood" from conception on. Most writers, including myself, focus on the parents' role in the development of many mental disturbances. In this chapter, I would like to examine the role of childhood leading up to prenatal conflicts and how these affect bonding between the new mother and her child. We will be looking at new mothers as post-treatment patients.

ISABEL

Isabel called me seven years after she had completed treatment for anorexia nervosa. She explained that she married two years ago and was eight weeks pregnant. When she came in, I asked her how she felt. She answered me with physical symptoms first.

"I feel like I'm always on a rocking boat, nauseated. I can't see or touch a raw chicken without throwing up. I'm fatigued, which is so unlike me since I've always been a high-energy person. I'm pushing myself to fight the fatigue."

"How is being pregnant affecting you emotionally?"

"I feel scared. I know that it will make me fat."

"Is it hard to distinguish between fat and pregnant?"

"It's impossible if they look the same. I feel bloated, full, awkward. My pants don't close and I'm sure other people are noticing."

Isabel was becoming increasingly agitated as she spoke. She reminded me of her talk when she was actively anorexic. "How have the last seven years been for you with regard to these kinds of feelings?"

"I've always been conscious of my weight, even a little nervous, but nothing you would call anorexia. Now I feel the intensity escalating and I'm scared. I don't ever want to feel like I did when I was sick." She paused and looked at me, becoming a bit tearful. "I want to have a healthy baby."

I realized she had some sort of treatment plan in mind for herself. "What would you like to do . . . here?"

"I would like to come in for the rest of my pregnancy, and maybe a little after. I think if I see you, you won't let me get crazy again.

There's too much at stake now: my marriage, my baby. My life's more complicated."

"Do you mind if I weigh you for the rest of your pregnancy just like when you were a teenager?"

She laughed. "Yeah, I suppose the whole drill is in order. After all, you have to make me gain weight again, probably beyond my wildest imagination."

I looked at her and nodded playfully. "Yup, probably about twenty-five pounds."

"Oh, great! And I came here voluntarily." The playful sarcasm in her tone was clear.

"We might as well start today, so please kick your shoes off and get on the scale. I'll give you two pounds for everything you're wearing, and another pound and a half to equal your basal (first morning) weight."

She looked relieved as she got on the scale and said, "So if I want to know my wake-up weight, naked, I can take off three and a half pounds from what the scale says?"

I nodded.

"Okay, here goes." She slid the weights over until the bar balanced. She stared at the number, startled. "One hundred and fourteen and a half—no wonder I feel fat!" She got off the scale and put her shoes on angrily.

"Isabel, you are five foot five inches tall and nearly at the end of your third month. With our subtractions, that takes your basal weight down to one hundred and eleven. I'm sure that your obstetrician isn't exactly thrilled with your low weight at the end of your first trimester. Perhaps I should give him or her a call so we can tell you the same numbers. Your delivery weight should be about one thirty-five—minimum. You do know the baby, placenta, and water weigh fifteen pounds?"

In a tone out of the past she nearly shouted at me, "That would leave me at one twenty after I deliver!"

I reminded her, "You're the one who said you want to do this right and not get crazy over it."

"Now I'm already crazy!"

"This is what you've been frightened of since you found out you were pregnant. I haven't really surprised you with anything I've said, have I?"

She drew a deep breath. "No. I guess I just wanted it to be you who told me. I won't be easy here."

"When were you ever easy here?"

She laughed. "I know, I just wanted to warn you."

Isabel limited her weight gain for two more weeks, until her doctor told her that she was two centimeters dilated and this put the pregnancy at risk. She reported this to me at our session the next day.

I felt a sense of jeopardy that I hadn't felt for years. Initially, I had been warned by colleagues that I was treating patients who might die. One psychiatrist said to me, "Steve, why would you want to have a practice that's almost a practice of suicidal patients?" I assured her that I didn't believe these were suicidal girls. I did however have meetings with internists and pediatricians to establish what health alarms would evoke life-saving procedures used on these patients to minimize that statistical 5–9 percent death rate we were aware of. This made me secure that I had plenty of medical backup.

Now I was faced with a secondary jeopardy. I had to talk my patient out of behavior that could cause a miscarriage which would terminate the life of her baby. This was a planned pregnancy by a couple that wanted a baby, so my talk and treatment might mean life or death for that wanted baby. For the first time in a long while I was doing therapy while experiencing the pressure and urgency of a new therapist who imagines that every word said or omitted could spell success or failure for the treatment.

When I had to learn the danger signs of anorexia nervosa, I consulted with my colleagues in internal medicine and pediatrics. Now

I have to consult with my colleagues in obstetrics and gynecology to keep the pregnancy process in proportion, and of course keep myself calm when there is no danger.

One of the issues that most anorexics struggle with is their perfectionism, and the feelings of guilt and inadequacy that accompany failure at high achievement.

I said to Isabel, "I know that you want this baby." She nodded in agreement. "How would you feel if you miscarried, or the baby was born with birth defects, knowing that your low weight was a contributing factor?"

Isabel began to cry. "I would never forgive myself!"

"I thought so, and I wanted to warn you of this possibility now, before anything happens. Babies are born imperfect when a woman takes 'perfect' care of herself during her pregnancy, and still mothers feel guilty. But if you could identify your own behavior as a possible cause, even if it didn't affect the outcome, you would suffer greatly." Isabel nodded again.

"Now there are three lives involved: your husband's, yours, and your developing baby's. Can you afford to let your fear of changing weight and shape threaten everyone's future?"

"But I'm so scared! Maybe I have no right to be pregnant?"

"Why don't I talk to you through your pregnancy, and I'll stay in touch with your doctor. Remember, you are doing something very generous. You are lending your body to another person so that it becomes the instrument of that person's development. When you have delivered your baby, you can take your body back. In the meantime, I'll interpret the changes that your body will go through so you won't be left alone with your old anorexic fears." Isabel looked relieved.

The next session was quite different in tone and pace.

Isabel came in and looked at me as if I had done something wrong. She sat down on the couch and pointed to her abdomen with her index finger. "Look at this!" She was almost shouting. "I'm at the beginning of my fourth month and I'm as big as a house! Not only that but I have all sorts of cramps; my bladder hurts—I go to the bathroom twenty times a day—my bowels hurt, and my back hurts!"

"Did you ask your doctor about these complaints?" I inquired.

She looked at me as if I was crazy. "When you're a woman lying on an examining table, with your legs in the stirrups, and the doctor rushes in, pokes your abdomen, invades your privacy in ways that make you want to pretend you're not there at all, you're grateful that all you saw was the top of his head and heard him say, 'Please put your clothes on and meet me in the consultation room.' You want as little to do with him as possible. And once you're in the consulting room and he tells you that your uterus is exactly the right size and everything looks fine, you just want to get out of there and not invite any further examinations of your body."

She was out of breath when she finished with her diatribe, which I'm sure was accurate.

I don't think that my answer came as a surprise to her. "Maybe we should be talking about how you feel about being on your way to motherhood."

Isabel looked confused. She stared straight ahead. After a short pause, she began, "I don't know. I don't know if I deserve to be a mother after all I did to myself years ago with the anorexia. I don't know if I'll be good for my child. I don't know if I can handle the responsibility, and I don't understand how I could be crazy enough to jeopardize my pregnancy with worrying about looking pregnant. After all, that *is* what I am—*pregnant.*"

"Isabel, when you were anorexic, you distorted society's crazy message to women to be nearly fat-free. Now you're pregnant and you're demanding that you become a perfect mother. It seems your pregnancy has brought out the kinds of fears you tend to experience when you go on to the next stage in your life. Leaving home for college did it last time. 'Going on,' maturation, separating from who you used to be becomes a terror for you. Growth scares you."

She was tearful but smiled amid her tears and said, almost in a child's voice, "But you'll be proud of me. I gained four pounds and my doctor said my cervix closed up and I'm not dilated anymore."

I smiled back with more relief than she knew. "I *am* very proud of you. It sounds like you are getting ready for the next stage in life we were talking about last time."

"I also heard the baby's heartbeat. It all feels so real now. I know it's not just about getting fat. I know that I'm making another person inside me."

ANNALYSE

Annalyse (Anna Lisa) was raised in a strict German family that ran a small-town department store. When she was eighteen, customers commented to her parents that their daughter at the cash register was looking strangely thin. Several of them asked her parents if anything was wrong with her. The parents hadn't noticed the fifteen-pound weight loss, which left Annalyse at ninety pounds at a height of five foot seven inches.

I treated her for four years, dealing with issues that centered on whether or not she was entitled to ask for what she wanted, or refuse what she didn't want. She had no language for requesting, demanding, or refusing. She could not do this at home, and when she began to date, a boy fondled her and she just sat still, tearful but quiet. She didn't protest. She stopped dating and began to lose weight. Annalyse was determined to be so thin that no one would find her attractive.

Toward the end of treatment, she had gained weight to one hundred fifteen pounds and was able to ask for what she wanted most of the time. Home was the most difficult place to do this since her family was dominated by her mother's mother, who spoke only German. Annalyse never saw her mother behave assertively to her own mother, so it was still difficult for her, without a role model, to be assertive at home.

At twenty-six, she married a tall, sturdy, gentle man. Jack was the son and partner of his father's masonry business. He wanted children as soon as possible. He was thirty-four and didn't want to be too old to deal with them as teenagers. He was a planner. Annalyse called me for an appointment when she was six months pregnant with her first child. She was twenty-seven and married eight months.

Annalyse was always shy and low-key. She came in, smiled, and sat on the couch. "How are you?" she asked, as if we had met the week before.

"It's been five years," I answered. "I'm fine, just a few more gray hairs."

"You look the same." She followed this up with a look down at her belly.

"You look magnificent in the bloom of pregnancy," I commented.

"Then I look a lot better than I feel," she said softly.

"How do you feel?" I inquired.

"Fat, ugly, defeated."

"Defeated about what?"

"I don't know." She shrugged her shoulders.

"Did you want to have a baby?"

She shrugged her shoulders again.

"At first I thought it would be okay," she said slowly. "I wanted a baby. I don't care if I never work outside my home again. You know, I grew up behind the counter of the store. Sometimes I miss doing the bookkeeping. I could do something like that on a part-time basis at home. So I thought that it would be nice to have a baby. Jack really wanted a baby soon. I told him I thought we should get used to being married first, so that lasted eight months. Wouldn't you know it? I got pregnant the first month. The doctor told me I was pregnant, but it didn't seem real until I started feeling all these strange feelings; my breasts got larger and started to hurt. Even my bra hurt, they were so tender. My husband thought they were terrific, but he didn't like it when I said I didn't want to be touched there because it hurt. I was always tired and you know how I like to get a thousand things done in a day. Now I just want to lie down and rest . . . and worst of all, eat. I've never been so hungry in my life! I could eat all day. So I know I'm going to become a permanent blimp between not having the energy to exercise and my gigantic appetite. Now my clothes are getting tight. I can't button my pants, even the ones I save for when I'm premenstrual!"

"How much weight have you gained in your six months of pregnancy?"

"Eighteen pounds—and now God knows how much I'll gain in the next three."

"Anywhere from seven to ten would be perfect, but I'm sure the idea terrifies you."

"Why do I have to gain any more weight? Don't I look big enough?"

"The last trimester is for the baby to gain weight so it's mature enough to survive easily when it's born."

"You're *not* going to tell me that the baby will gain seven to ten pounds in the next three months and I'm going to have a twelve-pound baby, are you?"

"No, Annalyse. I doubt that you'll have a twelve-pound baby, but for the baby to gain three or four pounds, your uterus needs to become larger to accommodate it. You'll need more amniotic fluid for it to swim in and your placenta with have to enlarge to feed the larger baby."

"Oh." She looked annoyed at my believable explanation but she rallied. "So none of that weight is *me*. It's my baggage, or the baby's baggage, or whatever?"

I nodded. She looked relieved. She continued to gain an adequate amount of weight until her delivery. The baby weighed seven pounds six ounces. A very cute, bald baby girl who became a blonde when her hair grew in.

When Annalyse's baby was just seven days old, she returned for her next appointment. She came with the baby in the carriage. I was surprised at her request to resume appointments so soon after delivering, but Annalyse did pride herself on her physical prowess. She wheeled the carriage in and sat down with her chin in her hands, looking depressed. I walked over to the carriage and fussed a bit over the baby, honestly praising her appearance and eliciting a smile from her. "She smiled at me and waved her fists," I commented with delight.

"That's funny, she doesn't do that with anybody else."

"Well, she's heard my voice for the last three months," I responded jokingly. "But you look unhappy."

She shrugged her shoulders characteristically.

"Come on, Annalyse . . . out with it."

Tears rolled down her face. "I think that she's going to like my husband better than me. He's more fun, more interesting, warmer."

"You're making a lot of plans for a seven-day-old baby," I commented. "All of these plans are hurtful to you. Do you know why you are making them?"

She became tearful. "It just feels like that's what is going to happen."

"Do you want that to happen?"

"No."

"Are you willing to accept that you have the power not to allow that to happen?"

"What do you mean by 'the power'? Do you mean, am I willing to do things that would change my expectations? The answer is, yes, I'm just not optimistic that it will work."

"Do you think that it's in your child's best interest to find you uninteresting?"

"No."

"Do you think that it is in your husband's best interest to be seen more positively—not equally—by your baby?"

"I guess not. I don't think that he would want that, either."

"So now we have some reasons for you to act toward your child in a way that will make her confident in you, see you as fun and warm."

She nodded.

"By the way, where do you think you developed these ideas about being uninteresting? Do you think it's because you married a man who's much more interesting than you?"

"No. You probably remember when I was eighteen that I always felt like that at home. I always believed my sister was more interesting than I was."

"Now you have a choice, a choice you didn't have in your own childhood. You are creating your own family. You can decide how you will be regarded by your husband and especially your children. If they admire you, that will be better for everyone. If they are contemptuous of you, that will be bad for everyone."

"So won't she see right through me if I fake the confidence?"

"We are believable to our children. Our consistent behavior is irresistibly believable. Children need to believe in their parents or they have no one to believe in."

"Even if I don't believe in myself?"

"If you behave as if you believe in yourself, and your children believe that behavior—and they will—their belief in you is contagious. You will begin to believe in yourself despite your previous self-doubts. After that, your self-esteem will rise and everyone will benefit."

Recovered anorexics who have difficulty with pregnancy and its accompanying changes in weight and appearance are usually in the minority. Most send me holiday greeting cards with family pictures, writing that all is well.

Postpartum: The Recovered Anorexic as Mother

What kind of mothers do women who have had anorexia as teens or young adults themselves make? The answer, of course, is all kinds. It all depends on how they were helped to recover from their anorexia, and how loving and supportive a marriage they have made. I have found that they make very good mothers, who occasionally indulge their children but usually come through to set limits as well. Remember, the victim of anorexia is often an unusually nurturing person herself.

If a pregnancy is filled with doubt and fear the way Annalyse's was, or presents other problems of self-esteem the way Isabel's did, postnatal therapy is advisable and sometimes the use of antidepressants (if the mother is not breast-feeding). Breast-feeding makes some women feel better and more bonded to their child. But for the more anxious mother, like the two I have described here, breast-feeding may make them feel too tied to their baby, while having their husband or mother give the baby an occasional bottle may lessen this anxiety. Each case must be considered individually.

Although no generalization applies to all those who have overcome anorexia, a surprising percentage choose to become dietitians, nurses, physicians, psychotherapists, or other nurturing careers.

The degree of recovery that people make from this disease varies. Some theoreticians proclaim that "One is always recovering, never recovered." To that I have to say, "Nonsense." I have seen many girls and women (nearly three hundred) recovered on follow-up by their own reporting, from three to fifteen years later. I have certainly been made aware of those who have relapsed from one to three times, sometimes requiring several hospitalizations. Percentages are hard to come by. Results of obtainable statistics vary from a 25 to a 35 percent recovery. This is not an encouraging range, but as families, psychotherapists, and psychopharmacologists become more sophisticated, less distant from, less afraid of, and less hostile to the victims of anorexia, we should see this range move to much higher levels.

16

HELPERS

THIS chapter is addressed, first, to the professional psychotherapist, and second, to those who would augment or assist the
mental health professional in the goal of helping the anorexic
recover.

When anorexia nervosa first drew attention to itself as a prevalent, as opposed to an extremely rare, disorder in the early 1970s,
few knowledgeable professionals were prepared to treat this illness.
My comments and anecdotes in chapter 14 were not meant to single out any one hospital as being undertrained or unorganized to
care for anorexics; none of us were.

My own work with anorexics began in 1970. I was lucky enough
to have a patient who recovered even though her therapist didn't
have any grasp on theory or techniques specific to her disorder.

By the mid-1970s, I was working with a half dozen girls with
anorexia and certain commonalities of their needs and features of
the personalities were becoming apparent. I described these in earlier chapters but will quickly summarize them again here:

—failure to develop trusting dependence on a parent
—turning inward toward self-reassurance when distressed

—development of obsessive personality traits
—development of perfectionism
—problems with feelings of emptiness
—lack of a sense of developing identity (or a negative identity)
—a weak sense, if any, of their own femininity
—remarkable ability in many cases to mask all of the above with charming, pleasing, outgoing behavior and success in school as well as social coping.

In 1978, Hilde Bruch, professor of psychiatry at Baylor University in Texas, published the first book on the subject of anorexia nervosa for the public, *The Golden Cage*. She turned to this subject after four decades of studying all manner of eating behaviors and disorders. In the same year, I published a novelized case study, *The Best Little Girl in the World*, after eight years of working with these girls and young women.

The victims of this disorder came out of the closet in the tens of thousands. They were searching for treatment, feeling very relieved that they were not "unique freaks," as they expressed in many letters to me.

At first, clinical psychologists and the medical profession were caught off guard and were even reluctant to treat these endangered, uncooperative patients, who didn't want to be patients. Professor Arthur Crisp of St. George's Hospital in London warned us all that the first task in treating an anorexic is to make her into a patient— to accept her status as a person with a mental illness.

Studies were commissioned, grants were created to look for genetic, physical, hereditary, psychological, and societal causes. Most of us agree, they all play a role.

A virtual subdivision of the health care profession developed with the speed and energy of a new industry to fill this vacuum. Unlike Alcoholics Anonymous, from the beginning these new groups stayed within medicine, psychology, and psychiatry.

Still, the diversity of treatment styles was extensive. Self-help groups sprang up, usually adjunctive to medical advisers. They were often started by mothers of girls with anorexia who could not find a place or success in conventional medicine and psychiatry. (See Appendix B for a detailed list).

Nutrition assistance groups and practitioners, usually licensed dietitians, encompass many specialists in this area who work with therapists, internists, psychopharmacologists, all conferring with each other and working directly with the patient.

In the last twenty years, the development of all these helpers is testimony to the stubborn power of this illness, and the army of professionals it takes to help an individual recover. If you are the parent, or the spouse, of someone with anorexia nervosa, you will read your health insurance policy only to find out how little of this is covered. The alternative to remortgaging your home is to substitute some of the professional services with family energy and redirection, as discussed in the chapters on family systems, reparenting, and others. Medical supervision is necessary to ensure physical safety. Psychological assistance is necessary for evaluation, diagnosis, and at least guidance, if not treatment. Clearly, the more professional services a family has access to, the more successful the outcome.

The self-help groups often have group meetings where specialists lecture. More important, families of victims can come to share their feelings about the afflicted member of the family without feeling guilty. Often strategies that have been helpful to a member of one family can be helpful to another family.

But self-help groups for victims themselves, groups that lack a professional leader, attract members who have a hidden or unconscious agenda: "I'll get everyone in the group to gain weight but me," or, "I'll nurture others but not accept help from anyone else." Sometimes I characterize these groups as "Eight therapists in search of a patient." Not a good idea.

The Nonprofessional Helper

Several traps await the best-intentioned helpers when working alone with an anorexic. This holds especially true for the non-professionally trained helper. I will call these traps "Worry love" or "Worry care" or "Need to rescue." They all develop out of feelings experienced by someone related to an anorexic through family, friendship, or institution (religious, school, college, team, sorority, etc.). Seeing someone that you care about starve herself, oblivious to her own endangering behavior, evokes a spectrum of feelings. They include fear, frustration, anger, guilt, hopelessness, and denial.

Fear is the most natural first response. When we see someone in danger, we naturally mobilize to help them. If they ignore our help, or refuse it, we become frustrated, and after repeated attempts to overcome their resistance we become angry at them. We think thoughts like, "She lied to me," "She ignored me," "She's insanely stubborn," "She thinks I don't know what I'm talking about," or, "How dare she ignore me."

After a cycle of anger we may feel guilty, see the person once again as "sick," become less judgmental about her eating behavior, and go through the previous cycle several times again. Eventually, depending on our relationship to the anorexic, we will give up trying to help, withdraw from her (unless we are her parents, and even then it happens), and regard her as hopeless.

Sometimes when one approaches the anorexic, she seems receptive to accepting help. She is talkative, appears open, even encourages her would-be helper by explaining she is changing her eating patterns. Since her mood seems friendlier, more pleasant, and her talk suggests that she is making improvement, the helper is encouraged, never noticing that the anorexic continues to lose weight or at least not to gain any weight at all. Most anorexics are irritable while gaining weight. They are usually in pleasant, even euphoric moods while losing weight. In this case, the helper is only too glad to deny that the weight isn't changing, or is changing downward, and may even believe that the change of mood portends weight gain. This response is known technically as "denial."

The nonmedical professional who is treating anorexia runs the risk, as a result of medical ignorance, of not being able to tell when an anorexic is in real danger due to slow heart rate (bradycardia), low blood pressure (hypotension), liver or kidney failure, or other physical malfunctions that can lead to sudden death syndrome. On the other hand, the helper may be frightened, even panicked, when the anorexic is not in fact in medical danger at all. The crudest rule that many who treat the anorexic use is a height-to-weight scale or ratio, usually: *Five feet tall=one hundred pounds.* Add five pounds for every inch taller and subtract five pounds for every inch shorter than five feet. There is an additional assumption based on several studies that once a girl or woman has lost her period due to malnutrition and low weight, she will have to weigh ten pounds more than the scale in order to regain her period. (The scale for boys is eight pounds +/– for each inch above or below five feet.)

This scale does not take into consideration the bone structure, frame, or what we call "surface" area of the patient, which makes it very approximate. Arguments about the time span of loss of the menstrual cycle (amenorrhea) and its relation to permanent loss of fertility vary, as do its relation to osteoporosis, the depletion of calcium from the bones due to estrogen loss. We equate loss of the normal length of menstruation within the cycle as a strong indicator of insufficient estrogen production, which will cause a variety of aging-related problems for women.

Many helpers operating outside a community of professionals may hear horror stories from the anorexic they are trying to help about their mistreatment at the hands of professionals and institutions. While none of us are prepared to say that no wrongdoing exists, even on the most professional levels in medicine, psychology, and psychiatry, we must remember that a feature of anorexia nervosa is "divide and conquer." In psychological terms, we call this "splitting."

Earlier, I referred to a leaderless group of anorexics as "Eight therapists in search of a patient" as a way of indicating that each member has enormous resistance to gaining weight but would like to see those around her do so for several reasons; she would maintain a competitive edge in the universal competition among women to be thin. She would also satisfy her need to feel nurturing by "helping" others, but not herself. I referred to a distinguished English psychiatrist, Professor Arthur Crisp, warning us that our first task is to make the anorexic a patient. So it is no small task for even a trained leader to take on a group of persons who would all like to lead but not follow, submit, or defer when it comes to the physical and psychological aspects and issues that are part of their illness, ranging from eating and weight to dependency, trust, identity, and femininity, among others.

The person who would lead such a group needs to be knowledgeable in the areas described above, and in addition will have to be the "nurturing structurer" of the group. A formidable task for an individual therapist, but exponentially enhanced by the group's "united resistance."

The leader of a group of anorexics is not a "facilitator," as group leaders often identify themselves, but may have to facilitate as part of his or her repertoire in guiding the group through issues that anorexics resist discussing. What needs to be encouraged within the group is not generosity (there's usually plenty of that in this group population) but having members willing to receive, depend on, and trust other members of the group.

In chapter 11, "Treatment Choices," I discussed one of the dangers of group therapy with anorexics: "symptom pooling," or the mutual informing by members of the group about the disordered and sometimes dangerous behaviors in which they are engaged. Perhaps the best way of avoiding the value of "peer-instigated behavior" is for the leader to list on the blackboard all the behaviors—from physical exercising to the use of laxatives, enemas, suppositories, emetics, and diuretics—which may be used by this group. The information is bound to leak out anyway surreptitiously among the members. It might be better for group members to hear it from the leader, along with all the dangerous side effects, emphasizing habituation and the potential problem of actual addiction to these behaviors and chemicals. This disclosure removes that precious conspiratorial secrecy when forbidden information is imparted from one peer to another. It also devalues the "recommended" behaviors.

Identity development is an ongoing, lifelong process for most of us. At different stages in life, different events and people can shift our sense of self to something larger and more positive, or to something smaller and more negative. During adolescence, despite the obvious rebellious behavior directed against authority, there are enormous opportunities for youth to incorporate ideas and ideals from authorities they trust. The most obvious negative examples of this can be found in cults, where late adolescents and young adults are seduced into the most obedient relationships and submissive postures by negative charismatic leaders. Why is it always the bad guy who is allowed to use charisma? Is charisma inherently negative or can it be used to create positive change? Is it our democratic heritage that makes us worried and even repelled by the use of charismatic influence for treatment in the mental health field? Perhaps we need merely to exchange the word "inspirational" for "charismatic" and we are on safer political ground. Whether one is leading a group in a psychiatric hospital, a free-standing outpatient setting, a day hospital, or a self-help organization, the quality or intensity of the leader's influence will be competing with the group's collective illnesses. Let's hope that quality contains competence, confidence, sensitivity, inspiration, *and* charisma.

We must never forget that anorexics are lost people pretending independence and confidence, pretending fullness of spirit and identity when they feel empty. They are secretly looking for someone who knows that about them.

The Helper's Self-Assessment

The would-be helper may not perceive himself or herself as needy, detached, a bully, timid, quick-tempered, inexpressive, unwise, or nonintuitive. But all these tendencies can be elicited by a suspicious, skeptical anorexic.

In defense of her illness, the anorexic (remember she defends her illness tenaciously) will look for evidence of such characteristics in a would-be helper, since most of us possess these traits to some degree. If she can zero in on one or more, she will behave in such a way as to exploit the trait until she can mentally dismiss the helper as undependable and untrustworthy. Once she has succeeded in accomplishing her goal, she will not surrender any part of the disorder she uses for her emotional protection.

DENISE

Denise (whom we have not met before) walked into my office and sat down glumly on the couch. She stared at the carpet, giving me no more than a momentary glance.

I opened our discussion, recognizing her discomfort, fear, anger, contempt, or all of the above, with, "Did you request that your parents bring you here, or were you *dragged* here to see me?"

Acknowledging my recognition, she looked up at me. "I was *dragged* here."

"Well, don't worry, you can only be dragged to see me once." I paused. Denise looked up, confused. "You would have to request a second appointment directly to me, or there would be none." She feigned relief that she would be free of me but became curious at the same time.

"What if they made me come back again?"

I smiled. "I would tell them what I just told you."

She seemed pleased that I wasn't intimidated or angered into bullying her in response to her rejection.

"So, what do you want me to say?" she responded, expecting me to reply, "Whatever you want to."

"I don't want you or *need* you to say anything. Your skeletal appearance, your thinning hair, your projecting pelvic bones, your protruding rib cage, and your discomfort at being in the same room with me all say a lot about you."

Now *she* began to look defensive and worried about the person she had just failed to intimidate. Perhaps I was a mind reader; then she would have no place to hide. Not even her silence could protect her from me getting to know her secrets. I increased her fear of disclosure when I focused on her face.

"In addition to your body communication, your face is very expressive."

She looked at me like a guilty wrongdoer, surprised and waiting to deny any accusation.

"What do you mean? Like my face is talking to you or something?"

"Sure it is."

"What's it saying?" she asked suspiciously.

"It's saying that you don't know how to cope with me, and you usually figure out what everyone wants or needs from you on meeting them. But I confuse you. It also betrays one of your best-kept secrets."

"What? What secret?"

"You know—the one about the wish."

"What wish?"

"The wish that someone will really get to know you and that they will know what to say to you, and even know what to do with you."

"Hah! I know perfectly well what to do with myself."

I smiled silently.

"What are you smiling about?"

"I was thinking about how brave you are, trying to take care of yourself when you don't know how to."

"But I *do* know how to."

"If you knew how to take care of yourself, you wouldn't be sitting here, starving amidst plenty, with thinning hair, a lower than normal body temperature, slow heartbeat, inferior musculature, and unable to concentrate as well as you used to."

Denise was startled by my directness and the probability that I might be correct about everything from her "secret wish" to my conclusions about her health.

She looked lost.

I added sympathetically, "I guess you would like to put a paper bag over your head for privacy now."

"Over my whole body." She smiled.

"Do you want to come back for another meeting?"

"I guess so."

"Is that yes?"

She slumped in her seat, took a deep breath. "Yes, I mean yes."

This is often the style of practice that I use in a first session with a highly resistant patient who tries to find neediness, frustration, impatience, and finally, of course, feelings of defeat in me.

Since I know more about her agenda and her illness than she does, I don't let her take charge of any part of the conversation in the session. I remain in charge. If I don't, I will disappoint her and she will dismiss me. I am steering the formation of our relationship to a point where she will come to trust me and eventually depend on me for emotional support. At that point I become more important than her anorexic voice.

Other Helpers

Parents are the easiest to dismiss because they are intimidated and fear the medical danger their daughter has placed herself in. Once frustrated, they can also become alternately bullies and quick-tempered. As they grow more confused, their gut wisdom and intuition about their child disintegrates.

With Denise, I was using an example of neutralizing the power of an anorexic patient, which applies to a therapeutic session more than an encounter between parent and daughter. This needs to be modified for parental behavior. Parents, unlike a therapist, experience feelings of responsibility, guilt, anger, and frustration toward their child. All of these can be felt at the same time or in the cycle in which I have presented them. These feelings greatly limit parents' ability to thwart the anorexic postures that emotionally "reward" their child.

To break the cycle of guilt that leads to feelings of anger at their child, parents usually need support and assistance. It is important to remind oneself that self-blame will not make a parent kinder or more helpful to the child. Parents need to be reminded that the loved child is a lost person who must be led, kindly but firmly, out of that strange forest we call anorexia. When the parent breaks the cycle of guilt, then the parent can parallel the therapist's style discussed above.

This concept is even more difficult to explain to grandparents. Grandparents are easy targets for resistance because they are unfamiliar with the day-to-day personality of the anorexic, unless they live in the same house or baby-sit for them often. They too become intimidated, and bullies, surrendering their intuition and gut wisdom when they make such well-meaning remarks as "What's the matter with you? You eat so little, you look terrible, like you're just out of a concentration camp! Are you crazy?"

Friends also can become easily intimidated. They are afraid of losing their friendship by angering their weight-losing friend, or saying the "wrong" thing and causing them to get sicker. After awhile, some friends follow a commonsense approach, state their concerns about their friend's appearance, and suggest that they should gain weight and get professional help. When this advice is ignored, friends become detached and often guarded toward the anorexic. These defenses are employed by friends to minimize the feelings of inadequacy and failure engendered by their friend's stubbornness and attitude (illness).

Friends need to remember that they are unlikely to "cure" their anorexic friend, that they are not responsible or able to help in this area. This will help them to avoid negative or fearful feelings about their friend. They should however avoid talking about their own dieting, or plans to lose weight—or, for that matter, any discussion of weight or comparing weight or figures.

Physicians often fall into a different trap. They are used to giving directions and expect patients to follow them. After all, that's why the patient comes to see the doctor—for a diagnosis, procedure, and directions. When the anorexic comes to see the physician, after the physician first rules out any medical condition that might account for the weight loss, he or she makes a diagnosis of anorexia nervosa. The physician then duly warns the patient what are the dangers to her health if she doesn't increase her eating and decrease her exercise activities. He instructs her how to become healthy again, and avoid becoming sicker, or even dying.

When the patient returns to the doctor several weeks later, having lost another six pounds or so, he is frustrated by the fact his sound advice was ignored, thus sabotaging his attempt to help her. As he becomes quick-tempered and detached, his next step is to bully her with all sorts of threats of hospitalization, nasogastric tubes, and anything else he can think of. All of this is understandable, but such an approach further alienates the patient.

Physicians need to diagnose and monitor the anorexic's health status via continual examinations of organ functions (heart, liver, kidneys, reproductive system, circulation, bone density, and blood values), blood pressure (no less than 80/50), and of course, weight, calmly reporting them to the patient. When examination results warrant it, the physician calmly informs the anorexic patient what steps or procedures he or she will have to take, including hospitalization. The physician may believe that he must "cure" the anorexia. In fact, the physician needs to limit his responsibility to keeping the anorexic out of medical danger.

In cases where medication is prescribed, the physician is in reg-

ular contact with the psychotherapist and with the psychiatrist prescribing medication.

Schools and Colleges

Until the last five years schools, especially colleges, did not feel
that students with eating disorders were their responsibility. And the
more they learned about the difficulties inherent in the disorder,
the less they wanted to look at the problem. After all, it would
require additional personnel, additional salaries, and possibly additional liability.

As early as the mid-1980s, I was involved with many student
health programs at northeastern colleges that were prescient about
these problems and changing parental expectations.

Recently, college programs have been set up to avoid some of the
traps that await would-be helpers. First, a series of tiers of investiga-
tion and inquiry has been introduced, beginning with a student
who believes he or she has identified someone exhibiting eating-disordered behavior. The student briefs the resident adviser, who may
make direct contact with the student or refer the student directly to
the dean (especially if the student is living in off-campus housing).
The dean then refers the student to Student Health Services for
diagnosis.

After the diagnosis, and depending on the degree of medical danger, the student's parents are notified to remove the student from
campus or the student is placed in a campus-recognized individual
and group health situation. The student is also evaluated weekly by
a campus physician who reports his or her findings to the dean.
Depending on the student's progress in gaining weight or continuing to lose weight, an administrative decision is made about whether
to allow the student to remain on campus.

The college campus, like the psychiatric hospital, offers helpers
a chance to work as a team where they can support each other and
avoid most of the traps I have mentioned above. A disadvantage of

the residential college treatment is that the student may be suffering from homesickness, or a separation anxiety from her parents. In
this case, all their efforts may fail because the student is unconsciously showing the need to resume living at home with her parents in an attempt to repair serious damage in the family system.

17

AN EXCEPTIONAL CASE

W<small>E</small> have been looking at the most frequently seen anorexics: adolescent, late adolescent, and young adult
girls and women. Aside from chapter 15 on "Pregnancy and the
Recovered Anorexic," we have not looked at the exceptional groups:
long-term or chronic women, pre-pubescent girls—and boys. Each
person afflicted with anorexia needs her or his own treatment, and
who is to say that only one kind of treatment will be the answer, if
there is an answer?

The Chronic Adult Patient

The chronic adult is the most difficult patient to treat. For purposes
of this chapter, I am not including the chronic adolescent. By "chronic," I mean the presence, for five years or longer, of strong anorexic
symptoms. I include disordered eating and digestive sabotage, exercising excessively, and maintaining abnormally low weight or fluctu-
ating to and from it. Mentally, this includes ideas that distort body
image (even further than society encourages it); anxiety and obsessiveness about trivial details of eating, elimination, and exercising;
and usually, but not always, a small, routinized daily existence.

There are many reasons why treatment is the hardest for people in this category. The most powerful is that they are rarely in conflict with themselves about their illness, which has become more of a natural way of thinking and acting for them. The anorexic's friends and relatives may not feel the same way, but she is inured to their disapproval, fears, and threats. She becomes a bit like the ninety-year-old woman who is scolded about her smoking. "What can you tell me?" she might ask. "These cigarettes will give me a disease— I'm ninety, so they'll shorten my life?" While this is a bit of a stretch, in contrast to the agitation her family might have gone through during the first few years about their daughter's anorexia—the criticisms, the death threats, hospitalizations, being dragged to treatment, threatened with restrictions about money and travel—those around her are all used up and she's still alive. She is living her life the way she is most comfortable and the original reasons for the onset of the anorexia don't matter any more. She lives this way by choice and is free of most of her "interferers."

Sometimes the anorexic has married and her husband has made adjustments to his wife's illness. It may even suit his own needs to overlook whatever shortcomings he experiences in himself by comparison. If she lives with her parents, they may have grown accustomed to "keeping" their daughter, even if she is ill. They are less lonely in their old age. Such acceptance by significant others is usually an adjustment on their part rather than a wish that the person remain sick, or in her patterns. What is missing in the chronic adult's life is an authoritative figure who could take charge of her and put her into treatment. At her age, even the law protects her from that happening. Most states demand that two psychiatrists prove "danger of *imminent* death" for commitment, which is usually for too short a time to matter, or to cure the illness.

Recently, a television personality in the Midwest was identified by her co-workers as being endangered due to her emaciation. They believed she was starving herself. They actually had her committed for several days. She was released, went home, did her last television show, and died of malnutrition despite the involvement of everyone around her and the law.

The principal difficulty in treating anorexia nervosa is that the patient is emotionally resistant to gaining weight, despite her intellectual understanding that she "ought to" do so. When this difficulty is compounded by the fact that she is no longer a minor and no one has legal or financial supervision over her, coercion is not viable as a method of getting her into treatment, even when it is clearly necessary to save her life.

When the ideas that have been listed above become ingrained over many years in an individual, they stop becoming an illness and evolve into her sense of identity. She may not be comfortable enough to admit this to others outside therapy, but nevertheless she does not expect who she has become to change.

Psychotherapy can be used as treatment only so long—especially treatment to change behavior and ideas that currently provide security. After awhile the patient becomes "therapy-savvy," and like one who has seen a dramatic movie over and over, remains unaffected by even the most intense moments. I am not suggesting that psychotherapy is entertainment, but it does require intensity and involvement. This in turn requires an experience with some novelty and freshness to be effective. Someone who has been repeatedly exposed to the standard accepted treatments for anorexia is not likely to respond to yet another exposure to them.

A special requirement for the adult, long-term patient is a therapeutic relationship that has a personal connection that exceeds previous therapies while maintaining realistic boundaries. The therapist who is capable of being more real, and more sensitive when he or she is talking to the patient, is the most likely to succeed. In this manner, the therapist becomes more valuable to the patient. She may be willing to try harder for change if she feels that the person she is allied with is valuable to her.

GRAHAM

Graham was twenty-eight years old. She developed anorexia when she was a freshman in college. She had been a horseback rider all the way through high school. Her affluent parents had traveled a lot and she also traveled on the riding circuit. She had platinum credit cards which she used liberally. But during her freshman year at college, her father suffered massive business reverses. He had to sell the four family horses, including Graham's, which she had taken with her to college. She began losing weight a month after she said goodbye to her horse. At the end of her freshman year, her weight had dropped from one hundred and fifteen pounds to seventy-two. She was five feet four inches tall. She had left a prestigious college during finals week and was suspended pending a review of a request for readmission.

Her father bought her a studio apartment on New York's Upper East Side. She lived unsupervised, and unaccompanied by relatives. Her parents and two sisters lived in Boston. Graham developed rigid patterns of eating and living in general. Every activity she did was prescribed by style and timing, from waking up at seven in the morning to moving her bowels at ten. In the evening she would eat a bowl of rice, one grain at a time. She did the same with string beans and peas. Dinner took over three hours to complete.

She applied to less prestigious colleges over the next three years. They all accepted her. She began a term at each, but stopped attending courses by the middle of the term.

When Graham called me for an appointment, she spoke in a mechanical voice, devoid of expression, intonation, or inflection. She came in dressed plainly but neatly. She did not make eye contact but stared in the direction of my face. Her replies were brief and guarded. "Yes," "No," "Three years," "Two sisters," were typical. I inquired about her guardedness.

"Do you always answer so briefly?"

"Yes."

"Do you feel attached to anyone?"

"My mother."

"Do you communicate with her more expressively than you do with me?"

"No."

"How do you experience this attachment to her?"

"It's just there. It's not great."

"What would make it great?"

Graham sat in silence. It was too dangerous a question to answer. It would bring up feelings that she didn't want to feel.

Graham came regularly to her appointments for six months in very much the same colorless fashion she presented at our first meeting. She had gained no weight. I offered her dozens of long, "long answer" questions, only to get short answers in response. Then she canceled several appointments one after another, so I asked her, "Do you want to continue seeing me? I don't get a sense of either improvement or change in your pattern of behavior, or even a relaxation of your guardedness toward me."

Her reply was slightly less stiff than usual.

"We both have invested a lot of time in this and I think it would be premature for us to abandon it at this time."

For Graham, this was intense though severely understated, but that was Graham. She made eye contact with me after the first year of therapy. This was about the same time that her speaking pattern loosened up and her answers to questions lengthened and a "Graham" began to emerge. It would be nearly two years before she began to surrender her low weight. Not until the third year would she indicate in a straightforward manner that her meetings with me meant something important to her.

"If I gain weight and weigh a 'normal' amount, do I have to stop seeing you?"

This came as a surprise to me, since Graham's style of communication would not betray any attachment or connection that she had toward therapy or myself. I also understood that this was an understatement, the second understatement she had made about seeing me.

She *was* forming an attachment toward me, but forbade herself to acknowledge it directly, either by stating it or by her style of relating to me, which was matter-of-fact and distant.

I answered her question carefully: "No, when you reach your goal weight, we just begin to work on all the issues that your low weight hides, or at least minimizes to you. The issues of your identity, dependency, trust"—she rolled her eyes—"attachments, and femininity."

"How could a *man* help me with my femininity? You can't be a role model. You can't know enough about women to guide or instruct me. I mean," she looked playful, "I bet you couldn't even tell me how to put on lipstick." She smiled, proud of the challenge she had put out to me.

"I suspect you don't have much of a sense of femininity. You are right, however: I couldn't teach you how to put on lipstick. But I don't think that's what it's about."

She looked at me, both puzzled and challenged.

"Then what *is* it all about?"

"Do you feel that you have more in common with other women your age, or that you are more different from them?"

She looked down for a moment. "I guess I feel different from them."

"How?"

"Other women are in couples or single. But most of them are interested in becoming couples, involved, or at least hooking up with someone of the opposite sex, or same sex. I feel neuter, nothing about that. I'm not a lesbian, but I can't see myself with a guy, either. I guess I'm literally out of it."

"How about non-romantic friends, platonic friendships?"

"Oh, sometimes I call a friend from my original college. I guess I'm a snob, and I didn't really make any friends after the first college, but I don't get together with anyone outside of my immediate family—and that's only when I can't avoid them."

"You don't like them?"

"No, it's not that. It's just that they'll get in my way. I mean, I have certain ways of doing things, at certain times. I can't say to them, 'Excuse me, I have to take two hours to eat lunch and it has to be at two o'clock.' So I stay away, except for those 'special' holiday occasions when it would hurt their feelings too much."

The second phase of therapy came when first I, then we, could talk about our therapeutic relationship—what happened between us when we talked to each other. This occurred during the second year.

When Graham came in, I asked her about her weight. She looked at me and said, "It's a little better but I don't like that because I feel like I've gained ten pounds. So I guess what you would call 'better' I'm not happy with."

"Are you aware that this is the first time that you looked at me directly while answering a question? In the past you have only looked at me when I was speaking, but not when you were."

She shrugged and gave me an embarrassed smile along with a playfully sarcastic answer. "Well, don't expect that all the time. I only have a few direct looks left."

During the second year of treatment, there was some progress with weight gain but her frequency of vomiting remained the same and her reclusive patterns did not change.

Graham would fail to show up for one-third of her appointments for several months at a time and then return to consistent attendance for awhile. After three years, she "slipped away" from treatment. I made several attempts to contact her, but she did not return my calls. Five years later, she called me from Washington, D.C., to ask me for a referral to a therapist there. I gave her several names but was pessimistic that her pattern would change.

In retrospect, I think we had begun to make some progress toward change and recovery, but the sheer length of time Graham had lived a life consisting of no responsibility, no connection to others, made her eating disorder the only structure in her life that she was organized around and could depend on. I couldn't compete with that. She never considered hospitalization, or any group treatment center, or medication.

Additional Stress Factors

When we talk about mental illness, we always include, along with family history, health, and family psychiatric history, *stressors* — those aspects of a person's life which discourage recovery due to the tension, hopelessness, or fear they produce. A major stressor for Graham was dropping out of college for ten years and feeling that she could not get a job consistent with her family background and expectations, or even social acceptance along the same lines. The extraordinary length of time she was involved in her illness, or its *chronicity*, was a second major stressor.

In addition to stressors, we look for *enabling factors* which would support the illness. Sometimes we see a spouse who is comfortable with a sick partner so his or her own deficits and problems can be overlooked as he plays the "healthy" one." He may cater to her every anorexic behavior and give her extra positive attention for it. Other times we find in families the need on the part of one or both parents to have a sick child to cling to, one that won't grow up, become independent, and leave a needy parent behind.

In Graham's case, we had a combination of enabling factors: a father who would never restrict her financially, a mother who would talk to her on the phone four times a day, and the structure provided by both to make the disorder inviolable — her own private apartment with the rent paid, no job required, no social or financial responsibilities to distract Graham from her disorder. The combination of stressors, of entering a world in which Graham felt like she had no place educationally or vocationally, no social network to return to, and the enabling factors which kept her safe within the walls of her apartment contending with no one, were a powerful set of realities to perpetuate her illness permanently.

I have seen patients Graham's age or older who have had anorexia nervosa for longer periods of time overcome it and go on to have successful careers and relationships. But they are less likely to succeed than the younger, less chronic anorexic. They all usually will need more time, up to five years. They will also need more frequent sessions, two to three (or more) a week, so that the therapist has a greater percentage of their time to compete with this major part of their personality. Often it is advisable to have their families come in at least occasionally, if they are available, to limit the stressors and the enabling factors as they emerge.

Nearly all diseases and disorders, both medical and psychological, respond better to treatment, and offer a better prognosis, when they are diagnosed and treated effectively earlier rather than later.

The Very Young Patient

At the other end of the spectrum is the very young patient, new to the illness and sometimes pre-pubescent, eleven years old or even younger. I recall two such patients, both eleven years old, making the same declaration, "I don't want to be a teenager!" When I asked each one why they didn't want to become an adolescent, they didn't know. A typical discussion would sound something like this one with Judy:

"I hate the idea of being a teenager."

"What bothers you most about it?"

"I don't know."

"Suppose I make my question a multiple choice and you can choose what aspects about adolescence scare or repel you the most?"

"Okay."

"Are you afraid of changes in your body shape? By that I mean the development of your breasts, hips, thighs? Are you afraid of having menstrual periods? Are you afraid of other people's expectations of you to act 'older' than you act now?"

She paused. "It's *all* of those. There isn't one good thing about getting older or growing up."

"Do you know any teenager or grown woman you admire?"

"No. My parents are divorced, my mother is miserable, and the kids in the eighth and ninth grade scare me with their makeup and their showing off for boys."

"So, you don't want to be a teenager because you don't feel like it's a good thing to be and you don't have any idea how to do it?"

"I guess you could say that. It's more than that, though. I think things are expected of teenagers. I don't want any more expected of me."

"You sound like a lot is expected of you already, or you're afraid of new and different things that will be expected of you as a teenager."

She burst out crying. "Yes! I think that a lot of things *are* expected, or *will be* expected of me, and I don't want to have to," she fumbled for the words, "produce them or 'do' them. I don't even want to look like one of them!"

"Judy, you keep repeating that you don't want the physical changes that come with being a teenager, and that you don't want to have to meet the expectations of others, perhaps new responsibilities, more advanced social behavior, and even romance and sexual activity. Maybe you have left one more thing out, and that is 'leaving childhood behind' before you are ready to."

"Well," she began softly, "I'm *not* really ready to do that either, as a matter of fact. I like being different. I like to play with different personality types." Here she looked at me mischievously. "Does that make me a multiple personality?" She giggled.

"No, it makes you imaginative—something that you don't have to give up when you become a teenager."

"Do I have to give up wanting my parents to protect me . . . sometimes? Or to expect them to comfort me?"

I smiled and suggested, "I think the high end of the age you can hope for that is toward forty."

She smiled and jumped up out of her chair. "Really! You're not kidding, are you?"

I shook my head.

"So, what's the deal? How can I start this change so that no one will notice and *expect* anything?"

"We can have your ears pierced."

She thought about that for a minute while she fondled her right earlobe, staring straight ahead. "Okay! Will my parents let me?"

"I'll recommend it."

Judy had her ears pierced. She slowly reentered school on a part-time basis (every other day) and gradually "tolerated" her place as an eleven-year-old, "Neither here nor there," as she put it. She became interested in acquiring more earrings. She then became interested in developing "my own look," as she put it. We met for two years, during which she rapidly recovered her weight and became positive about the physical changes she was going through as her biological adolescence proceeded. She proudly announced to me the arrival of her first menstrual period, as well as other changes.

I met with both of her parents and we discussed ways that they could help Judy recover. Both stressors and enablers are more powerfully represented as parents with the very young (and not so young) anorexic. Each parent, since they were divorced, was asked to find a support person to discuss their own neediness and anger with. They would try and eliminate these topics with Judy. They would praise her for all positive steps she took—socially, cosmetically, academically—whether they represented something that an older girl would do (but not dangerous) or even something a younger girl would do (which would cause her social penalties). As pre-pubescent children and early adolescents vacillate between childhood and its fears, and middle to late adolescent dress and behavior, it's important both to be supportive and to warn them of the consequences of either extreme. Criticism of Judy would require that delicate diplomatic balance of softness without weakening the behavior in question.

Luckily, Judy's parents both loved her more than they wished to settle old marital grudges, so they cooperated with the program.

Three years after the onset of her anorexia, Judy was symptom-free and had developed a group of friends.

18

THE NURTURANT-AUTHORITATIVE

PSYCHOTHERAPIST

So far, I have discussed the role in treatment of the family, parents, hospital staff, and nonprofessionals as helpers in assisting a person to recover from anorexia nervosa. There are many ways a person can recover from anorexia. Some recover without any assistance at all. Some recover by falling in love. There are those who have recovered because of a marked change in their lives, whether it has been centered on people or geography. There are those who have recovered out of fear, or sheer inspiration. All of these groups combined, however, make up a small percentage of those who develop the illness, and a smaller percentage of those who make a total recovery, estimated at between 25 percent and 35 percent. The aspect of treatment I would like to elaborate on here is the role of the individual therapist, an aspect I term "nurturant-authoritative psychotherapy."[*]

The nature of anorexia has not changed in the two decades since it became apparent that the disorder affects one out of every two hundred and fifty girls between the ages of eleven to twenty-two,

[*] This topic is explored at more length in my book *Treating and Overcoming Anorexia Nervosa* (New York: Warner Books, 1982).

while the recovery rate remains low and the number of those afflicted keeps rising. One positive change is that public awareness and early detection have reduced the number of anorexics admitted for hospitalization, while outpatient individual psychotherapy, along with medical, pharmacological backup and nutritional consultation, has emerged as the main form of treatment.

When I worked with inpatients at New York's Montefiore Hospital in the 1970s, a colleague of mine, Preston Zucker, a pediatric gastroenterologist, would say to patients who averaged sixty-five pounds on admission, "It's my job to keep you alive, but it's Steve's job to get you over this, so work with him closely." Back then, it always seemed the issue revolved between life or death. Today, the battle is tilted between recovery or chronicity, a lifetime sentence for the afflicted.

If we understand anorexia nervosa as a security-controlling obsession which becomes the main characteristic of the personality, and we understand that the personality is most affected by its own inner rules, then we need ways to lure that personality away from the rules that govern it. We must understand that these inner attractive rules do not create real security.

If the therapist can both structure a relationship that makes that personality open to new emotional possibilities, and at the same time create a connection that offers relief from the endless self-reassurances inherent in obsessiveness, then we have a strategy for recovery.

The question of how these "attractive, obsessive" rules fail to provide real security is crucial for us to understand how to undermine the value of these rules to the anorexic. Once we have clarified the value of these rules and where they fail these victims, we can develop a dialogue that will produce the trust, dependence, and attachment that is necessary to undermine or diminish the victim's attachment to "the rules."

When I use words like "trust," "dependency," and "attachment" as part of a therapeutic relationship, I make many therapists uncomfortable. Inevitably, such questions arise as, "What are the boundaries, with regard to physical contact with the patient, time limits on meeting, place of meeting?" The answers are the same as for other patients, although what is required of the nurturant-authoritative therapist is more talking on the therapist's part; the role is closer to one of teaching about life and feelings with the patient, who may have an impoverished vocabulary in this area.

The therapist provides support and "coaching" when the patient is trying out new behavior that involves the feeling of risk and requires flexibility on her part. It is often up to the therapist to fill in the "empty places" that the patient complains of, which we call "deficits." These deficits represent missing information and coping skills in one's personality. This therapeutic relationship style seems more "real" because it is more interactive between patient and therapist. It still maintains the same structural boundaries (length of meeting, place of meeting), and of course this is a talking therapy as opposed to a physical contact therapy—"therapeutic" touching, holding, etc.

In an age in which less parenting is available to children because both parents usually work—and often in high-pressure jobs, with long hours—talking has a parenting component that many schools of psychotherapy have difficulty accepting. Today, perhaps the most difficult concept to accept is that in addition to the nanny, the therapist will be required to act as a surrogate parent, rather than a professional person using professional tools to "treat" an illness the way a physician would. Indeed, the therapist assists in the development of an adolescent the way a full-time sensitive parent would if she (or he) stayed home.

In the past, the population of psychotherapists was almost exclusively male. But psychotherapy has now partially shifted to the social worker, who is more often female than male. The feminizing of psychotherapy needs to be accepted as a positive change, rather than attempting to imitate a male model that was largely medically oriented and useless to many patients.

The Therapist's Medical Knowledge

Although I have deliberately aligned "medical" with "male" negatively as a style of psychotherapy, as being too mechanical (by this I was referring to procedures, research, and mechanical style of the therapist), I do wish to stress that without a working knowledge of medical knowledge in areas affected by anorexic behavior, the therapist is lost.

Treating anorexia nervosa has been viewed negatively by psychotherapists because

—They don't see themselves as patients
—The patients don't want to get better (gain weight)
—It is one of the few disorders that involves deadlines (to gain or stop losing weight)
—The patients place themselves in real medical danger by their behavior and this angers and/or intimidates the therapist
—Weekly concrete evaluations may be made by parents and physicians, placing additional pressure on the therapist

A basic working knowledge of the medical norms and dangers posed by starvation (restricting of eating) and weight loss include:

—Understanding when low weight is statistically at a dangerous point for the patient
—Understanding norms for blood pressure, body temperature, heart rate (beats per minute)
—Understanding blood values: potassium, protein, and iron, among others
—Understanding visual abnormalities, e.g., lanugo, thinning of scalp hair, nearness of veins to the surface of the skin, skin wrinkles that can be misinterpreted by the anorexic as fat tissue

Nonmedical therapists are not expected to measure or evaluate such bodily functions, but they should be in contact with a primary care physician on a regular basis to help both of them make therapeutic and medical decisions about the patient. These decisions will include: whether or when she should be hospitalized, whether adding nutritional compensation is necessary, and whether they think the patient will cooperate.

This collaborative relationship between the primary care physician and the psychotherapist will protect the patient, the physician, and the psychotherapist. Sometimes the psychotherapist will have to alert the physician about an observation that suggests the patient may be in medical danger. Sometimes the physician will have to relieve the therapist's fears that might interfere with treatment behavior by reassuring the therapist that the patient is *not* in medical danger, despite the therapist's worries. Clearly, it is in both the physician's and the therapist's interests to work closely together for the best results with the fewest misunderstandings—communicating directly with each other and not through the patient.

Countertransference

One can easily understand that in treating anorexia nervosa the therapist needs opportunities to protect himself—or herself—from getting either overly concerned or underconcerned about the patient's safety and recovery. These are similar to the worries that the patient, parent, or spouse experience. In a sense, the therapist's bind is how to be really empathetic and attractive to the patient, while he remains professionally/emotionally safe to make therapeutically wise decisions.

Since anorexics are always testing the emotional strength and confidence of their therapist, he or she needs to possess real confidence and technical competence when working with the patient. The battle of wills is between the anorexic ideas, rules, and trust, and the therapist's belief in his or her own rules and trustworthiness. So, we have a seeming paradox to resolve: How to treat someone authoritatively, while at the same time the patient perceives the therapist as a nurturing person. This is of course a dilemma that most parents face constantly while supervising and taking care of their child. So there is a parenting element in the treatment relationship between therapist and patient, the therapist being experienced as the "good parent."

Nearly all anorexics deny their need for nurturing. They often exhibit a hysterical, tyrannical demand for obedience by others. This is the anger their unsatisfied needs for nurturing have produced. The therapist has to deal with this tyrannical behavior and comfort the hostile patient. To accomplish this, the therapist has to see through the superficial repelling behavior as a defense against fear of the patient's neediness. I once asked a patient, "Why are you so afraid to trust me? I suspect you are tempted to."

"If I trust you and depend on you, you'll suck all the air out of the room and I won't be able to breathe."

Alice was talking metaphorically about the way she experienced her mother's behavior toward her when she thought her mother was "nurturing" her.

"So when I'm 'nice' to you, you try to push me away or behave as unlikable so I'll stop 'tempting' you to accept my care?"

She shrugged and nodded in reluctant agreement.

"So, when you've pushed me or anyone else away from you, you have the space to continue your obsessive ideas about your fat, the backs of your arms, your stomach, your thighs, your waist, and so on. In addition, you can analyze yesterday's eating, today's eating, whether you should starve so you can eat 'normally' at tonight's party. Then you can go on and see if you've exercised enough, check your limbs for firmness, reflect on whether you could have pushed yourself harder. What a fascinating mental and physical life! I'm sure it provides a lot of growth."

Alice looked thoroughly scolded and ashamed. She kept staring down at the floor. I waited out her two-minute silence. Finally, "So what am I supposed to do?"

"I am going to presume you have asked an honest question and give you an answer. First, you have to stop pushing for space between yourself and others, especially me, because I won't respect your mental privacy. You do terrible things with that privacy. It's isolation. It's stagnation. I, unlike your mother, will not 'suck all the air out of the room.' You will have to get used to the idea that others have something positive to offer you and sometimes you can only receive it when you are vulnerable to them. I am not suggesting that you become indiscreetly vulnerable to the world, nor does it mean that you become sealed off from the world."

"Do you know how terrifying this idea is to me?" she asked.

"Do *you* understand what is at stake if you don't do this? A lifetime of stagnation. You will have no personal life. You will continue to turn inward until all you do is come home from work, exercise until you think you 'deserve' to eat, then measure out your food on a food scale, use special-sized plates, eat slowly to enjoy every bite of your tiny portions, and go to sleep or watch TV until two in the morning. Is that what you would like to see yourself doing for the rest of your life?"

This young woman was twenty-two years old and had just graduated from college. She was living with her parents and looking for a job, so she could move out and away from their constant harping on her eating and exercising habits. Their relationship was a roller coaster of continuous anger and guilt.

Working with Parents

Parents of anorexics often are fearful of doing or saying the wrong thing. They fear that this intrusiveness will cause her to eat less and lose more weight. After awhile, the parents experience mental "abbreviating" (see chapter 4) and simply feel fearful when their daughter is present even if the context of the situation does not involve eating.

Mental health professionals sometimes underestimate the resourcefulness, or potential resourcefulness, of the parents of an anorexic and suggest that they remove themselves from her eating and exercising behavior. Unfortunately, again through the abbreviation process, this leads to a disenfranchisement with their roles and undermines their confidence in parenting. This dynamic increases the child's isolation and she becomes increasingly sick. Inept or insensitive parents won't help the situation; but retreating and abandoning their roles as parents will almost always accelerate the disorder until it has reached a chronic state. At that point, everyone begins to believe that the patient will be sick for life or until the disorder kills her.

Often parents will need a therapist that they can see without their daughter, whose presence would intimidate them or sabotage the strategies for coping in specific situations. They will probably need continuous support from a therapist in order to battle the persistence of both their daughter's behaviors and postures toward them. By the end of the first year since the daughter (or son) developed anorexia, the family system has evolved into what we designate as an anorexic family system.

If one therapist treats both the daughter and the parents, he or she will be suspect to both parties and confused by the discrepancies in the reports presented by "each side." While it can be done, it is usually easier and more effective to use two therapists.

The therapist who works with the parents has two major goals: First, to help the parents confront the conflicts between each other, especially parents who do not have the ability to adopt new behaviors toward their child; and second, to nurture and support the parents so they don't inadvertently turn to their daughter for emotional support or even approval. That kind of interaction fuels the anorexia. The parents' therapist is almost like a good grandparent figure in this therapeutic family arrangement.

The therapist who works directly with the identified patient acts as a "good-powerful" parent figure, who guides, advises, counsels, and interprets the patient. It is quite an active role for any therapist to take on.

Deficit Building

Soon after the anorexic gains weight, or while that is happening, issues of dependency, trust, identity, and femininity (or masculinity) need to be introduced by the therapist. The patient is ashamed of her deficits, so very often the therapist must begin with a "teaching talk." This teaching talk opens the patient to the experience of "receiving" from another person and readies her eventually to talk about topics that she doesn't normally allow herself to talk about. Remember, she despises her own feelings of neediness and denies them to the best of her ability. Like the parents of the patient, the therapist cannot look to the patient for approval or support that he or she is on the right track. There is a risk here that what is being said by the therapist is not specifically what the patient needs to know at the moment. But the therapist can do a reality check by asking, "Do you follow me?" or, "Is this hard for you to hear?"

One might criticize this approach as grandiose on the part of the therapist, to think that he or she knows more than the patient, but if we look at the relationship that the patient has with her family, we usually find submissive, needy, or disengaged parents, in relationship to their daughter, especially since she became sick. Most anorexics know that they are lost, despite the phony confidence they display outside their family. The confident therapist is a welcome relief. This therapeutic posture will, however, make the patient uncomfortable, since she doesn't know how to behave in a relationship where she is not either in charge or at least manipulating the other person. It is a good idea to tell the patient that she will not know how to react to the therapist for the first few months and to let her know that this is normal for this extraordinary situation. Any bit of support that the therapist can sneak past his overly pseudo-independent patient will reduce her resistance to further change. It will also help her realize her deficiency in the area of trust.

It is important for the therapist to comment on the patient's behavior and nonverbal communications, especially facial gestures that give clues to the patient's feelings. This accomplishes two goals: It tells the patient she is being validated and therefore she doesn't need to rely on her false, manipulative self; and second, it marks the beginning of a new cluster of identity messages that she will incorporate.

"Therapist Shyness"

Twenty years ago, I was invited by the teaching hospital with which I was affiliated to present a talk in the department of pediatrics on "Physician Shyness." The talk was to deal with the difficulties physicians experience when they have to examine young patients in rectal or genital areas. I spoke about the need to explain the genital area being examined to the patient, and that if a schematic drawing wasn't available, the physician should clearly give the patient the medical label for his or her genitalia and the components of its makeup.

An experienced physician raised his hand. "Couldn't I just say that I have to examine you 'down there'?" (To this day I don't know if he was trying to help me or sincerely meant the question.) I responded with, "Do you have a part of *your* body that you call 'down there'?" The rest of the staff—mostly women—burst into laughter. I continued, "It is important to demystify both the body and the mind to someone who needs help." If a physician is to examine a child old enough to understand the use of the words, a drawing of the genitalia could be made and the words that make up the organs can be comfortably stated by the physician. These words for the male include: penis, testicles, scrotum, foreskin, urethra; for the female: labia (inner and outer will do for the Latin "minora" and "majora"). If the problem includes the clitoris, I recommend it be identified as the "tingly-buzzy" place. The distinction between the urinary tract and the vaginal canal is useful to girls and they usually accept this information with healthy curiosity.

Many anorexics are missing as much information as the child

who is being examined by the physician. To assist the anorexic in "owning" her sexuality and womanhood (if her age is appropriate), the therapist must be able to explain and discuss sexual anatomy and behavior under appropriate circumstances, when necessary. Television's Fred Rogers could do this for three-year-olds because he was playful enough and kept the explanations within their understanding. If the therapist is shy, it indicates to the patient that this is a forbidden area to think about. Remember, anorexia nervosa victims have demonstrated that they have distortions and are ignorant about their body's proportions. Imagine how many concealed areas of ignorance and distortion have to be uncovered before they can accept a healthy attitude toward their bodies and bodily functions, especially when feelings of feminine identity are involved.

Often the safest place to begin a discussion is questions about the menstrual cycle: regularity, length of periods, cramps, and the patient's attitude to the whole experience. Again, if the therapist is shy (or ignorant) about these issues, he, or she, will limit the patient's trust and therefore the effectiveness of the therapy. Alternatively, when the patient senses that the therapist, whether male or female, is comfortable with these basic feminine issues, more comfortable than she has been, then such issues can launch the kind of trusting dependency that is necessary for the therapist to compete with the anorexia for the patient's security system and comfort.

The therapist's approach to such a sensitive topic is critical to its success. It is helpful to warn the patient that this topic may be uncomfortable to discuss. Often I tell my patients that for awhile I might have to do 90 percent of the talking, especially if I am dispensing information. Most anorexics are vastly ignorant about their bodies and their femininity and will feel a bit embarrassed at first just to hear the information. I also reassure them that this same information will become less loaded, even boring (as I am repetitious). I try to do this in a playful manner to lighten the tension. Feminine issues should be dealt with intermittently, otherwise they become too ponderous for the patient. Changes in the patient's behavior that indicate progress include the following:

— Her facial expression (while the therapist is explaining) changes from a blank stare, indicating discomfort, to occasional eye contact and nodding to indicate understanding
— She breaks her silence and asks questions about herself
— She brings up problems her girlfriends (real or disguising herself) are having, gynecologically or sexually

Many late adolescent anorexics (eighteen to twenty-four years old) feel hopelessly inadequate socially and sexually. This accounts for their fears that going away to a residential college will expose their immaturity. Even if they don't go away to college, they often shy away from girls their own age when the topic turns to boys and sex.

I believe one of the tasks of treating anorexia nervosa is to deal with these issues with the reassurance that unless there is a history of child molestation, rape, or incest, the patient can be mentally and emotionally "caught up" within a year. This is not to state that sexual activity is necessary, just having the emotional choices available.

KATERINA

I was recently reached by phone by a former patient whom I had treated for anorexia from the ages of eighteen to twenty. She "slipped away" from treatment after she gained weight and her eating was relatively normal, though rigid. That was ten years ago.

I picked up the phone to hear a cheerful "Hi, this is Katerina Andersen. I saw you a long time ago. Do you remember me?"

"Yes, you lived in Connecticut and wanted to be a model." She was relieved at my recognition but her tone changed abruptly to an angry sadness.

"I would like to come back to see you if that's all right."

"Of course it's all right. Do you want to tell me what prompted your call?"

"Yes. I'm thirty years old and I'm still a virgin! I never develop much of a relationship with any guy and I don't know why."

Katerina was a strikingly pretty girl, so I knew she had to be sabotaging herself romantically.

"I guess we never finished all the issues we should have covered when you were in treatment."

Her tone became apologetic. "That was my fault. I know I dropped out. Maybe I didn't want to address 'mature' issues. Well, my leaving treatment was a lousy idea because now when I get really frustrated, I find myself staring at toilet bowls and throwing up. Something I never did before."

Katerina returned to treatment. She declared that her goal was to overcome her sexual impairment, or deficit.

"I don't know anything about my own body! When other girls, I guess I should say women, talk about their experiences, I have nothing to contribute to the conversation. I just don't think of myself as a woman." She was tearful. "I didn't want it to turn out this way!"

"I guess we'll just have to catch you up on your knowledge of your body, your sexuality, and your arousal. We'll have to catch you up on men's sexuality as well."

"Then you don't think I'm hopelessly sexually retarded?"

"Oh, I think you are retarded in your development, to use your word. I also regret that we didn't attend to this ten years ago, but we'll have to catch you up now. This talk may be embarrassing at first. Are you up to it?"

"I'll have to be. I can't stand being like this."

In subsequent sessions, we discussed sexual anatomy. I asked her to look at her genitalia with a mirror in the privacy of her bedroom or bathroom. I described what she would be seeing, and asked her to come in with any questions. We talked about hormones, menses, fertility, and sexual activities.

After a half dozen sessions she asked me, "Am I supposed to be comfortable with giving a man oral sex? I hate the idea and I think it's disgusting."

"The specific sexual acts that people engage in vary by mutual preference," I assured her. "These acts cannot be gratifying if one partner—you, in this case—finds them disgusting. Most of the women I've spoken to about this prefer not to do it, even though some do it anyway. Today, there is a pressure on women to be sexually professional in 'servicing' men. I hear this from college women as well as high school girls. It must be a leftover from the seventies when all of this started. Back when feminism was at its most radical, men took advantage of equality of the sexes and many women picked up half the check on a dinner date because men whined they were being used as a meal ticket. They complained that if men and women are equal, then they have equal sex drives, and if the man pays for the dinner, the woman has an obligation to sleep with him. I always told women that when men go through menstrual cycles, become pregnant, and give birth, then they will be equal. Until then, they could hold doors for women and pay the dinner bill.

"But to answer your question specifically, no, providing oral sex for a man is not a requirement and not a criterion for sexual normalcy."

Katerina looked so relieved at this answer, her whole body went limp. "Oh . . . are you sure?" I just nodded. She stood up and smiled.

"You mean never, I never have to do that even if I get married?"

"Two people should do what pleases them both, not just one of them."

"So I won't be a freak if I never do that? A man won't leave me because of it?"

I thought I'd reduce the drama at this point. "No, you never have to do that. No one who cares about you will ever leave you over it, but please don't tell the fellas I told you that."

Katerina giggled. "What a relief!"

"Is it possible that because you have been worried about this activity being inevitable in a romantic relationship, from the first meeting with any man, you have acted more like a pal, one of the guys, someone who doesn't behave flirtatiously or seductively?"

"I don't know how to act seductively, or even if I do, it feels too scary."

"I guess we should be talking about acting seductively as a rehearsal for you to 'try yourself out' with a man when the opportunity arises and you are interested in attracting him."

Some might argue that this is more the work of a sex therapist, or even a "social coach," than a therapist. Earlier, I mentioned that treating anorexia requires teaching, guiding, counseling, as well as interpretation and insight therapy. This is one of those examples. In sessions that followed the one cited above, Katerina came in with questions about how to cope with specific situations I answered them, or at least explored the choices and possible outcomes.

One day she called me frantically and explained that a famous elderly photographer had met her and invited her to his house on eastern Long Island for a "weekend shoot."

I responded uncharacteristically, "No, he's attempting to exploit you sexually. Tell him you would be happy to meet him at his New York City studio for a shoot."

Apparently my response was more emphatic than I was aware of. She came into my office several days later and said, laughing, "You practically shouted at me when I asked you if I should go to his house. I was so relieved. I just said to myself, 'Well, that's that.' I did call him as you suggested, and he said to me, 'I think maybe you are too shy. Do you know what erotica means?' I said yes. Then he said, 'I wanted to take some pictures of you for my private collection. I hadn't planned to show them to anyone else.' I thought, well what good will that do me if I want to get jobs as a model? Thanks for making it so simple. I was so relieved when you said no! I stopped obsessing and actually forgot about it."

Although this is an extremely directive approach in treatment, it isn't really different from requiring that the patient change her eating patterns in order to gain weight.

The Nurturant-Authoritative Approach

Sometimes the issues are not as clear as the need to gain weight or change eating patterns. The therapist clearly takes on more responsibility in treatment when he or she makes a direct recommendation. The passive, inquiring, more analytic therapist takes markedly less responsibility and avoids the kind of real interpersonal conflicts that have to be resolved if he or she is "wrong." The absence of real interpersonal conflicts is often a characteristic in the family life of the adolescent, or in the upbringing of the adult anorexic. The development of these conflicts in therapy, and working them through in therapy, is part of the treatment in nurturant-authoritative psychotherapy. In the example cited above, my "demand" that she not go to the photographer's weekend studio was viewed by Katerina not as domination but as protection.

In nurturant-authoritative therapy, the "authoritative" component functions as protection more valuable than that offered by anorexic behavior. Of course, the therapist must be on solid ground when he or she makes an authoritative intervention. The therapist must also be able to distinguish between meeting the patient's needs with this kind of intervention as opposed to his own need to dominate (value system, excessive fearfulness for the patient, etc.).

When a patient is hospitalized, an "authoritarian" structure is assumed. With the shortening of hospital stays, which limits the therapist's ability to do reconstructive psychotherapy since this takes quite a while, the outpatient therapist must put in place some of that structure in the therapeutic relationship. The outpatient therapist is doing therapy with a patient who can quit by just walking out the door or terminating the relationship with a phone call.

The nurturing aspect of the relationship is the other side of the "trust" coin. This conveys to the patient that the therapist cares and that caring also creates more security than anorexic behavior. It is based on a very old parental expression, "I'm doing this for your own good." If the child believes it either at the time it is said, or after the child gets over feelings of anger and resentment, the trust between parent and child remains intact. If this feeling has always been in place, then it would take an exceptional event or circumstance to make the child vulnerable to anorexia (see chapter 19).

The personality of the therapist is critical in creating a reparenting, or nurturant-authoritative therapeutic relationship. Today, most therapists I have met are more comfortable behaving in a sympathetic, nurturing style than they are with the authoritative posture. In effect, this makes the patient experience the therapist more like their parent.

Combining the two components or postures creates a powerful alliance of treatment that some therapists are uncomfortable with. I have been asked at many conferences, "How do they ever leave you? How can they ever end therapy?" My answer is usually, "The same way my own children grow up and leave home." Their security base may be established by others, but eventually it is incorporated by the individual herself (if she is allowed to by non-needy caretakers) and she leaves home base to strike out on her own. It begins with adolescence, where the child may sometimes strike out with rebellious behavior and alternately stay close to home for security. It evolves into adulthood, where the two extremes are balanced and children call their parents for advice, or visit them out of their historical love for each other. In the case of therapy, I usually get holiday greeting cards and pictures of new babies from former patients. They outgrow the intensity of those first few years in treatment and their attachment to me.

The nurturant-authoritative therapist has to be comfortable with the patient's attachment and at the same time maintain boundaries so that he or she won't be manipulated or controlled by the patient's attachment, either personally or professionally. The patient is made aware that she is not up for adoption by the therapist. The therapist doesn't find the patient on his or her doorstep, suitcase in hand.

Like most career choices, psychotherapy is chosen by those who like the task, and feel they have the desire and aptitude to succeed. Obviously, some career choices are not made for these ideal reasons. In any case, even within psychotherapy, as within medicine, different personalities make choices to specialize in a certain field. Some therapists reading this chapter will choose, or already have chosen, to work with these particular patients; others will prefer different types of patients. All therapists' choices involve some degree of specialization, even if a therapist has "multiple specializations." Treating anorexia nervosa requires substantial specialization and years of experience, which unfortunately cannot be obtained overnight.

As I have already stressed, treating anorexia nervosa as a psychotherapist must also involve a degree of familiarity with the medicine related to it: weight norms for a patient's height and frame, nutritional blood values, daily and weekly caloric intake requirements, norms for healthy functioning of the vital organs, liver, kidneys, heartbeats per minute, blood pressure, gastrointestinal functioning, reproductive system, electrolyte norms, and others specific to each case. That is why we don't treat anorexia without an internist or primary care physician's continuing collaboration. We may also need a psychopharmacologist, if psychiatric medications are necessary; a gynecologist, if the patient reports reproductive system abnormalities; and an endocrinologist, if their metabolism is abnormal. Sometimes an ear, nose, and throat specialist is required if the patient experiences pain or bleeding from vomiting.

Finally, in the requirements for the therapist who treats eating disorders, I must include a strong stomach.

19

ANOREXIA IN THE
NONDYSFUNCTIONAL FAMILY

U P to this point I have used illustrations of various family dysfunctions to show how they can sabotage the development
of the emotional trust and dependency necessary to maintain security and stability for a predisposed anorexic.

There are however certain other circumstances, having nothing
to do with family or other relationships, that will unfortunately put
in motion the same forces of mistrust and failure of dependency.
These forces will lead to the same results, and the final form of the
disorder will look like all the others.

The Impending Death of a Parent

LESLIE

Leslie was one of two children. Her brother was three years older.
He was an intellectually gifted child who talked early, walked early,
and when he began school, teachers were hard-pressed to find challenging tasks for him. He was also cheerful, generous, and even-
tempered. Leslie on the other hand was discovered to have several
learning disabilities, among them dyslexia, and was visually astig-

matic, so it was difficult for her to read without shifting lines. From the beginning, she did poorly in school. Her parents had her tested by a thorough educational psychologist who gave them the bad news that Leslie had severe educational impairments that would hamper her chances for scholastic success, no matter how hard she tried.

Leslie's IQ had to be measured by a test that would not be affected by her eye-to-brain impairments. The test indicated that she tested in the superior range. The irony that this bright child, with less vigilant parents, would come to think of herself as dull, inadequate, and develop powerful feelings of inferiority, was intolerable to her parents.

Her father was a successful attorney who had to bring work home in addition to his daily office work. But each evening after dinner, he spent three hours helping Leslie do her homework and study for tests. If the result was a D, he praised her for it. If the result was a C, they had a mini-celebration. His enthusiasm was apparent to Leslie, and while she knew her brother was getting As, her father's enthusiasm drowned out the scholastic norms for her. She trusted his judgment, felt his love and appreciation of her, and his pride in her. She grew up with high self-esteem and developed none of the negative feelings she might have had without his powerful energy and support.

When she was fourteen, her father was diagnosed with intestinal cancer. The family's upbeat reaction was that he would fight this and possibly defeat it. Most of the time, Leslie blocked her father's "chronic illness" and its consequences from her thoughts and feelings. Occasionally, it would flash through her mind like a bolt of lightning, as she would put it, but she dismissed it as fast as the thought crossed her mind. However, it did leave a residue of fear, which subconsciously began the process of lessening her dependence upon him, and lessening the expectation that her father would always be there. Gradually, Leslie began rather reluctantly to become more independent, telling herself, "It's up to me now."

There was no loss of love, affection, and camaraderie between them, but it was laced with a subtle fear and sadness.

During the eight years of the father's illness, the cancer spread to his lungs and his increasing debilitation became too obvious to be denied by any member of the family.

"No cancer, no nothing, was going to stop him from attending my college graduation. I wanted to cry when I saw him being helped out of the car and handed his crutches, but I didn't. I remembered he was the person who cheered when I got Ds in school," Leslie said later.

At the end, he was put on a respirator which forced his labored breathing. Leslie and her mother and brother stood around the bed. The mother was at the foot of the bed, facing him. Leslie believed he couldn't go on like this another minute. All the family members nodded as a silent vote was taken by the three people who loved him most.

"I told the nurse to turn off the respirator. His chest stopped its violent, tortured rising and falling. He breathed slowly on his own for less than a minute. He locked eyes with my mother until he was gone."

Leslie was smiling even as the tears streamed down her face.

"He looked so peaceful. It was over for him. I cried for a year. I cried on buses, walking down the street, God knows what people thought of me. I couldn't stop crying. I was accepted to graduate school and I didn't know how I was going to function. My mother suffered her own grief, and my brother, at twenty-five, became the man of the family and did everything he could do for me. Nothing helped. One day I looked in the mirror and decided I was too fat, something I never thought about before. I was always regarded as pretty, and at five foot four and a hundred and twenty-five pounds, I was always satisfied. I started to lose weight. I exercised until I thought my heart would pop out of my chest; at the same time, I restricted my eating. Altogether I probably ate about six hundred calories a day, I stopped crying.

"I would go on to school. Soon my crying disappeared. The starving and the exercising saved me. I became oblivious to all other feelings except those related to eating, exercising, and weight. I never had a goal weight in mind. I just never wanted to cry again, so I kept it up. My mother and brother begged me and yelled at me to stop losing weight. I could barely hear them. Didn't they understand how important this was to me? Well, soon I ran out of weight, in their eyes, anyway. My mother and brother took me out of school and put me in a psychiatric hospital. The eating disorder unit was powerful. I mean, it was unthinkable not to eat enough, and impossible to exercise. It was like a friendly prison. I entered the hospital at eighty pounds. I had lost forty-five pounds!"

Leslie smiled with pride.

"I cooperated with them. The faster I gained my weight, or as they put, 'reached my goal weight' of a hundred and ten pounds, the faster I could get out of the hospital—where I would lose the weight I had gained. It certainly was *my* weight."

When Leslie came into treatment, my scale said she weighed ninety-two pounds. She smiled, but her smile quickly changed to fear as she said, "My mother's going to stop the money and put me back in the hospital again!"

"Ninety-two pounds means that you've lost eighteen of 'their' pounds, as you put it earlier," I told her. "I think that you're much too thin, but you're just in for the first session. Your present weight does not put you at risk, but if you keep losing weight or maintain this weight, it won't do. We will meet twice a week and I will weigh you twice a week, with no weight-falsifying tricks, of course." She nodded. "And if you can gain from one to two pounds a week until a minimum of one hundred and five pounds is reached and maintained, I can help you deal with your father's passing without needing all this 'anorexinailia' to stop the tears."

"Okay, okay. I don't want to have to go back into that hospital and miss at least a term of graduate school." Leslie paused. "I *am* in graduate school. That's pretty neat." She nodded her head with a combination of self-satisfaction and gratitude to her father for all those nights and cheers he gave her.

"So I guess you'll do this because they'll be 'his' pounds and your pounds this time."

"How did you know I was thinking that?"

"Easy call."

"You're different from the people in the hospital."

"They were a big help even though you didn't like them. They got you here on time. I wouldn't have taken you at eighty pounds."

Leslie and I talked a lot about her father's illness and the supporting role he played in her life. At my request she brought in her family album and we looked together at pictures of this happy family. As the pictures brought us closer to the present, his deterioration and surrender to the disease became more pronounced.

It was an unusual course of therapy. There were no complaints about any family member, only praise. It was obvious that the support was genuine rather than a refusal to avoid conflict. At one point I asked her, "Don't you ever get mad at your father for leaving you?"

She smiled and nodded. "Yeah, sometimes when I'm alone, I look at the sky and shout at him for leaving me."

Leslie continued to gain weight; the first two weeks at one pound per week. The third week she gained three pounds, scared herself, and lost them in the fourth week.

"Now that you have proved that you can still make your weight go down, how about picking it up two pounds this week? I figure you owe me one."

"And him," she added.

Leslie gained the thirteen pounds I requested in fifteen weeks. She wasn't menstruating yet. I was concerned with her low estrogen levels. In consultation with a gynecologist, she was put on birth control pills.

Her low estrogen levels would inhibit her body from using calcium to build bone density, a process that normally ends in a woman's early thirties and can lead to osteoporosis—the breakdown of bone structure that brings about frequent fractures and pain, along with a continuing shrinkage of all the bones. Normally, this condition affects women in their sixties and older. But I have seen anorexics as young as twenty-two with osteoporosis due to depriving the body of estrogen through malnutrition, in some cases as early as the age of eleven.

Leslie's weight recovery in outpatient psychotherapy was far from typical in its progress. I praised her for her efforts in defeating the fears that gaining weight engenders in anorexics.

"Well, it wasn't easy," she said in mock complaint.

"I didn't think that it would be. But after all, you have two advantages that most anorexics don't."

"And what are those?"

"Not to take away any credit for your bravery and determination, but to add credit to your family's good mental health, you must never forget that even though your father's death, and the eight years of your getting ready for it, contributed to your becoming sick, it was his life devoted to building your strength and self-esteem that was our greatest weapon."

The next week, Leslie brought in letters her father wrote to her when she was away at college. She read parts of them to me. She wanted us to meet, so she could begin her recovery.

She continues in treatment. Her weight remains stable at one hundred and seven. We deal with her anxieties for her future, her current romance, and getting used to feeling better.

For Leslie, anorexia was a hiding place created by the constant emotional pain of losing her father. Luckily, it was treated within the first year and a half of onset, before the disorder would erase the memories and values she held. If events hadn't moved so quickly, and without the support of her mother and brother, her personality would have become entrenched in all the characteristics of those who have been sick with anorexia for years.

Serious Physical Illness

Years ago, medicine was extremely antiseptic to the point of dehumanizing patients once they crossed the Admissions desk. The patient was separated from family and placed in the hands of doctors. This was of little comfort to adult patients, and terrifying to pediatric patients. Fortunately, much has changed, especially in the areas of obstetrics and pediatric protocols. Husbands are often included in birthing courses (if they are willing) and present in the delivery room to be of moral support and assistance. This patient-family involvement amid the doctors in the hospitals has expanded to pediatrics, which is most important because when children are placed in a hospital away from their parents, they feel abandoned and terrified. They also make inferences about the event of their hospitalization. Some of these inferences include:

1. My parents can't take care of me anymore. They are "surrendering" me to strangers, where I can't be protected—no matter how much they embarrass me or hurt me.
2. I am not safe and have no one I can count on.
3. I am dying and will never see my parents again. I have something terribly wrong with my body.

Such inferences by a child could lead to the unconscious conclusion, "It's up to me, I can't depend upon others." This is one way the personality can begin to build up defenses that will eventually result in the character development described earlier outside the influence of the family system.

Chronic physical diseases may pose danger, pain, or impairment that can be interpreted by a child to mean she is not safe and those around her are unable to "protect/cure" her, or him. Another example of this can be seen in the case of John in chapter 4. We can look at a spectrum of symptoms, from allergies to asthma to diabetes to cystic fibrosis. Unfortunately, in many cases the child's inference is true.

Chronic physical diseases, as well as permanently impairing injuries such as loss of vision or loss of part or all of a limb, can cause changes in the family system. When such a change occurs, it is important to seek counseling to maintain the family's health despite the illness or injury. It would be an error not to recognize the impact on the entire family should one member be chronically harmed.

Frequently, the best intentions of other members of the family can backfire, causing guilt, anger, and confusion. When one member of the family changes, or is changed by events, all members are changed.

In many cases, the illness may "defeat" its victim, and she may develop a disorder like anorexia to escape its impact. Diabetes is most likely to trigger anorexia or bulimia. It has built-in tools to facilitate dangerous weight loss, which may prove very costly.

JILL

Fourteen years ago, I treated a sixteen-year-old diabetic anorexic who deliberately reduced the required dose of insulin so that her body would not be able to metabolize the calories she was eating. Instead, sugars remained in her bloodstream, removed by her kidneys and finally eliminated in her urine. She was eating but losing weight. The side effect from this practice was kidney damage, which if continued would result in renal collapse and death. Other side effects could involve blindness, the loss of limbs, heart failure, and other crippling or lethal pathologies.

When Jill was referred to me by a diabetologist, he indicated that she had attended programs at institutes for diabetics, but, as he put it, "She is a tough one. No one has been able to make a dent in her behavior. Sooner or later it will kill her. See what you can do."

Jill, a skinny five-foot-four girl who weighed in at eighty pounds, cheerfully explained, as she tossed her long ponytail back and forth, "I have a small frame, you know." She was implying that I could consider this fact and not the weight on the scale. Jill still had a pretty face, despite her low weight, and was using all the charm she could muster to discourage me from confronting her.

"You have a pretty face and lovely long, but thinning hair." (The "thinning" was my warning that the confrontation was coming anyway.)

"Thank you." She smiled politely.

"How old were you when you found out that you had diabetes?"

"Thirteen." Her smile disappeared.

"What does a thirteen-year-old girl think and feel when she is told she has a disease and there's no cure and it's dangerous?"

"She feels like an angry freak who's always going to have to live and eat differently from everybody else and it will kill her anyway!"

"What does she do?"

"She tries to forget about it and eats anything she wants—extra sweets especially."

"Then she is being mad at her body for its illness?"

"She's mad at her body. She's mad at God. She's mad at her family because she is told it's genetic, which means somebody gave me these lousy disease genes."

"You switched from 'she' to 'me.'"

"I try to stay away from 'me' and this crummy disease, with its crummy injections and high blood sugar, low blood sugar, and 'dangerous' warnings. Do you know how many times I've heard the word 'dangerous'? Millions! I don't give a damn about dangerous!"

"I don't believe you," I said, half-smiling sympathetically.

"You don't believe me? How could you be my therapist if you don't believe me? How could I trust you?"

"I believe most of what you say. I don't believe you when you're trying to fool yourself. Do you want me to?"

"How do you know when I'm trying to fool myself?"

"When you say things that are impossible for a sane person to feel but wish they *could* feel."

She stared at me, puzzled. I wasn't intimidated by her. I wasn't mad at her. I wasn't fooled by her. I *was* interested in Jill and her story. She nodded her head in surrender, with a hint of a smile.

"So, Mr. Mind Reader, what am I supposed to do about this disease? How *am* I supposed to feel about it?"

"Maybe we should start with what you *shouldn't* do with it. You shouldn't hide from your fear of it and you shouldn't use it as a baseball bat to bully your parents."

She looked mildly insulted. "I don't use it like a baseball bat and I don't bully people with it."

"You hide from it with your insulin purging, your anorexia, so now you have two baseball bats—diabetes and anorexia. I bet your parents are afraid of you all the time. I bet they walk on eggshells around you. That's easier for you to deal with. You feel tough and fearless and, of course, numb."

"You make me sound like a monster!"

"You like to feel like a monster. It gets out your anger about having the disease, it keeps everyone worried about you on two fronts, weight and blood sugar, so now you can be tough instead of scared, and lost to yourself and to them. I think that's a good choice. I'd rather feel that way if I were you."

She looked at me, bewildered. "So, who am I?"

"That's a good start."

"What do you mean?"

"I mean, you're tired of pretending that you know what you're doing. You're mostly tired of pretending to yourself."

"So?" she responded glumly.

"So, you're ready to get off your own case. You're ready to accept help, which has always been repugnant to you."

"And *you* are that help?" with a note of sarcasm.

"You like to test the strength of others around you who would be authority figures to find out if they really have feet of clay, and I enjoy listening and watching you test."

"You make me feel younger. I don't get it."

"You *are* young. I'm going to give you a chance to stop bluffing."

"How are you going to do that?"

I shrugged my shoulders, raised my eyebrows. "I guess I'll listen to you, talk to you, guide you, and manage you."

"Hey, that's a lot of control. Are you on a power trip?"

"No. I'm on a responsibility trip."

"I thought I would hate hearing anything like the things you're saying to me, but I like them. You're a confusing person."

"Ah, confusion is the first step to change." I smiled.

"Speaking of confusion," I went on, changing the pace of the conversation, "I want you to take a blood sugar reading now."

She looked shocked. "Why?"

"Baseline. I want to see how much you screw yourself up with all this."

"But I don't have my glaucometer here."

"I have one."

She looked nervous but resigned. When we were finished, we waited for the digital readout on the glaucometer. It read "High," which meant over 300; 125 was the top of the normal range.

I looked at her. "You know what that means?"

"Yeah, it means I really screwed up."

"How long have you been screwing up?"

"Two years."

I nodded solemnly.

"We will begin every psychotherapy session with a blood test. Then we will discuss what the reading means, for better or for worse."

"But you're a therapist, not a doctor," she protested.

"I am the only person who may be able to stop you from destroying yourself unless we lock you up."

"Okay, but this will make me gain weight—all the extra insulin."

"We are not talking about 'extra' insulin, just enough insulin. Remember, we are going to help you live without both baseball bats, anorexia and high blood sugar."

"I'll feel disarmed without my 'baseball bats.' "

"I'll help you find better ways to protect yourself without hurting yourself."

She cocked her head in mock suspicion. "You sure?"

"You wouldn't ask if you weren't sure of the answer."

Jill's case is not unique. Researchers have suggested that more than half of insulin-dependent diabetics have eating disorders, ranging from compulsive overeating to bulimia to anorexia.

Adolescents who develop juvenile diabetes often react over time by becoming angry at their bad luck and act out by breaking all the safety rules. The most obvious rules to break are those relating to eating patterns and insulin control.

In Jill's case, we worked together for two years. First, we took away the privacy of her symptom by my "policing" her blood sugar and teaching her how to express her feelings about having diabetes, with all its social drawbacks at events like pizza and especially beer parties (yes, the underage adolescent engages in beer parties, whether we like it or not), and the requirements for monitoring her blood sugar during what should be a carefree day spent with friends.

When Jill's symptoms were replaced with talk, they gradually disappeared. I helped her to accept her anger and let it diminish to a point where even though she might feel it occasionally, she would not act on it. She maintained normal blood sugar levels, as well as a normal weight, until we terminated the therapy.

Eight years later, I received a phone call from Jill.

"I just wanted to call you to let you know that I'm married, and have two healthy boys, *and* I'm still 'good.' You know what I mean. Thanks."

Often a healthy family can have an individual member attacked by a destructive event. This can lead the person to develop a symptomatic style of coping with it. She (or he) may exclude the rest of the family from "interfering" with the emerging symptom by retreating from them. This in turn puts in motion dynamics that can change a healthy set of family relations into an unhealthy family environment, full of anger, suspicion, guilt, fear, and diminishing communication.

Whether it is self-help or professional help, the goals here are slightly different in that they consist of maintaining family health and not letting the "event" destroy a healthy family climate.

20

INCEST VICTIMS

AND

ANOREXIA NERVOSA

s there a connection between incest and anorexia?" I have
been asked this question frequently. The answer is,
Sometimes. The problem with both the question and the answer
is the assumption that the majority of anorexics should be regarded as having been abused by a family member. When this experience has taken place, it does of course damage the anorexic. It
causes her to wonder about repressed memories, suspecting members of her family, adding to the problems her illness has already
created for herself and those around her. I have found that the
ratio of those molested as children and incest victims with anorexia is approximately one in five—not so different from the figures
for the general population.

Perhaps the more appropriate question might be, "Does incest
have a significant effect on the anorexic making her experience a
special subcategory of this illness?" I believe the answer to be, Yes.

Incest victims—or "incest survivors," as they call themselves, and
we should do likewise—have survived one of the most damaging
experiences possible, one that causes the greatest harm to developing normal mental, emotional, sexual, and interpersonal relationships.

The most common and intense effect on a child who has been a victim of incest is her feeling that "There is no one out there to whom I can turn for physical and emotional protection. *There is no one I can depend upon or trust.*"

When a child is deprived of the security of trust and dependency, as we have seen, she will turn to obsessional and anorexic defenses. The more intense the provocation to turn away from others, the more intense her defenses, and ultimately the pathology of her disorder.

The death of one or both parents is a tragedy that adversely and intensely affects a child's development in the areas of emotional and interpersonal relationships, and creates permanent fears of abandonment. Under these circumstances, such a child is also a candidate for obsessional disorders and anorexia. But this child can be partially compensated for her loss if grandparents, aunts, and uncles take over as primary caretakers and offer love along with the care. This in no way immunizes her against developing such disorders, but the chances for recovery will be greater. In contrast, the young incest victim, from her experience, has become "trustproof," or immune to developing trust toward another person.

The abused child will sink deeper into layers of mental defenses and ideas, which will make "compensation" for her original damage unacceptable. These defenses may include: amnesia or dissociated states, self-harm and self-abusing relationships, multiple personality disorders, and of course, eating disorders (and this list is far from complete).

When a patient comes into treatment for anorexia nervosa and any of the above-mentioned disorders, we term this "dual diagnosis." To treat dual diagnosis patients successfully requires more skill on the part of the individual therapist or individuals involved, usually involving more than one mode of therapy and many years of treatment. Even with all these resources in place, the outcome is uncertain.

The incest survivor who has developed anorexia is initially going to be the most difficult to treat. The work of the therapist is to reach, connect, develop a trusting alliance to begin the treatment process.

DONNA

Donna was twenty-one years old when she came into treatment. She was five foot six inches tall, weighed ninety-two pounds. Her pre-anorexic weight was one hundred and twenty-four pounds.

In addition to restricting her eating, Donna ingested Ipecac, an emetic that induces forty-five minutes of painful vomiting. It was easy to imagine that she had been an attractive young woman at her original weight. Now she looked drawn, pale, her facial features enlarged by the absence of any tissue between her skin and bones. Nevertheless, she was dressed seductively. Her smile was that of a posing model. Her skirt was short and she would occasionally slide down on the couch a bit, then readjust her position so that her skirt crept up several inches. Her panties were coming into view. Her low scoop-neck top showed a bit of bra and more of her breasts than would be regarded appropriate by most people.

I introduced myself and asked her how long she had been trying to get thin. "For about two years," she responded in a matter-of-fact tone. She had seen two therapists before me and there was no doubt she had answered these questions before.

"As a child, have you ever been sexually molested or raped by any member of your family?" I asked mildly.

She looked shocked, but after a moment responded in a loud voice, "Why did you ask that?"

"Were you?" I persisted.

"How could you tell?" She looked at me incredulously.

"When you come to meet a psychotherapist for the first time, and you display as much underwear and flesh as you are doing, you are trying to tell me several things: you worry that you won't be found interesting or valuable to me if you don't seem sexually interesting; or in the past you have been sexually exploited and you are testing me to see if I, too, will exploit you. If I *do* respond to you with sexual interest or advances, you're on home ground. It means you are physically 'used,' but you're used to that, whether you like it or hate it. At the same time, you are emotionally on guard by not trusting me and avoiding being disappointed."

"But what if my slip were showing and I didn't know, then you are really insulting me with all you've just said?"

"I don't think your example compares with what I just said, but I think that you have been sexually abused as a child or early adolescent. Am I mistaken?"

She tapped repeatedly on her right knee with her index finger. After several seconds, she noticed how high her hem was. Then she quickly pulled her head up and examined her chest. She looked at me sadly, shrugging.

Donna started to cry. "I guess"—she choked a little—"there *is* a lot showing. All those things you said—are they true?"

"Am I mistaken?"

"No. A lot has happened to me." She put her face in her hands and cried some more. Then she looked up at me. "It's my fault, right?"

"No."

Her seductiveness was gone. She adjusted her skirt and top. She seemed like a young, innocent girl who had been wronged, abandoned, powerless.

"I don't know whether I want to be so thin that men won't want me, or to get even with other women by being thinner than they are. I just know I can't stop trying."

"Trying to do what?"

"Trying to lose more weight. If my weight stays the same, I have a fit. If it goes up even a half a pound, I'm crazed."

"Who was the first woman you ever wanted to get even with?"

"First it was the girls in the eighth grade. That was a low-key feeling. Then one day I was watching my mother look at herself in the mirror. She was checking out her stomach. I didn't say anything, but you could tell she was worried about her weight. Her skirt was tight all across her pelvis. I grinned, I could feel it, but I knew she couldn't see me. That was the day, the day before my sixteenth birthday, I promised myself I would make her feel weak-willed, old, and fat."

I decided to support her expressed rage.

"You sound very angry at your mother. I'm sure you have lots of reasons."

"You bet I do! She sold me out. She allowed him to do things to me that I could not repeat to anyone!"

"Did she see these things? Are you sure she knew what was going on?"

"No, I don't think she ever saw these things, but she should have known that they were going on. My father is a drunk. She would leave me alone with him for long periods of time. He was slow and careful at first. He told me not to tell anyone. When he figured out that I wouldn't tell anyone, then he started doing weird things to me that hurt!"

She stopped herself. Her vulnerability was wearing out. Her need to let that frightened and angry little girl out was relieved. She stared at me for a moment in disbelief.

"I can't believe I just said all that to a man. How do I know you're not one of them?"

"Because I told you to cover yourself up."

"Yeah, no man ever did that except the assistant principal of the school, and when he did it, he looked at me like I was a whore. You didn't even look annoyed with me when I was showing you. I guess I was kind of 'flashing' you."

"I guess I should have told you before," I said playfully, "you will be allowed no sexual abuse here, even when you ask for it."

"Wow! That was the weirdest thing anyone ever said to me."

"I said it in a joking tone, but you will be confused here when I don't give you the response you are used to. Sometimes you'll be confused, sometimes you'll get angry with me."

"What happens if I get angry with you?"

"Nothing, we can work it out. We resolve the conflict between us."

"I've never done that with anyone before. I've never seen my parents do that. When they fought, they fought until one of them walked out of the room, or the apartment."

"What is *never* at stake here is the relationship, only the issue we may disagree on. I don't stop liking you because we argue and you don't stop coming here because you're angry at me."

"Then we're trapped."

"Not trapped—safe. Safe from abandonment, safe from fear."

"I don't know what that feels like."

"You'll be awkward while you learn what it feels like."

"You're scary."

"I think that for you, not knowing what to be afraid of is scary."

"I always know I'm afraid of becoming fat."

"Convenient."

"Are you making fun of me?"

"You know how to live in fear, a state of hyper-alertness. If things seem okay, you get uncomfortable. Sometimes you have to create danger for yourself. You might even have to generate pain for yourself. Do you know what I'm talking about?"

"How do you know this? I'm not saying you're wrong, but I never told this to anyone and I don't even understand it myself. Sometimes, a lot of times, I think that I'm crazy."

"Sometimes you *are* crazy . . . unreasonable, mentally chaotic. We'll have to work on fixing that."

"What do you mean? How could that be 'fixed'? You're either crazy or you're not."

"Is worrying about being too fat when you are nearly a skeleton crazy?"

"No, it *is* important."

"Starvation *was* important in the beginning, as a weapon against your mother. Now it's obsolete, out-of-date, meaningless, and part of that old familiar feeling of fear and anger; but they aren't attached to any real ideas anymore."

"So why is it all I think about all the time?"

"Because you have learned—and for good reasons, at one time—to stay emotionally alone. When you are not open to take in the thoughts and ideas of others, your own supply of ideas shrinks like your body until there are fewer ideas repeating themselves in your head with greater intensity."

"So I have to give up my fear of fat, my pain, and my anger?"

I nodded.

"That's impossible. No one can do that!"

"No one can do that without the help of another person."

"I don't believe people can help each other . . . only hurt each other."

"There's no doubt that your life has taught you that in the past, but what if the future could be different from the past?"

"How?"

"What if I could help you?"

She looked annoyed. "If nobody can help anybody, then how could you help me?"

"I never agreed that 'nobody could help anybody,' I just agreed that was your life experience. Other people have different life experiences."

She looked a bit agitated. "And *you* are going to be my different life experience? You expect me to believe that?"

"Not at all, at least not for the present. All I expect you to do is to show up for your appointments."

"See, that's what I mean. 'Appointments.' This is an office, you are a therapist. I mean, you're not planning on adopting me, are you?"

"No, I'm not planning on adopting you. I am planning on helping you. This is a room; whatever happens in this room happens between two people. It also happens between you and yourself."

"What does that mean?"

"When you think something, or even say something aloud in an empty room, it doesn't feel more real. When you say something about your feelings or ideas to someone you trust, you have made a declaration that has traveled from your mouth to *your* ear as well as mine. That changes you, a little at a time. That makes you and your feelings more real to yourself."

She looked at me curiously.

"You think that's really true?"

"Yes, but each time only a little changes."

"When will I notice a change?"

"I can't give you the exact date, but in six months you should see some difference in how you view yourself."

We were on safe ground now, away from eating and weight. She was not in charge and not engaged in any contest for power or seduction.

"You're doing very well in coping with a man you just met, in a manner you usually don't engage in."

She smiled, then caught herself enjoying the compliment I gave her for her personality, not her desirability. I thought she felt disarmed for a moment, vulnerable to trust. If this happened too often, it might unravel her defenses, which protected her from the pain of incest and weakened the defense of anorexia.

"Well, it sounds interesting," she said almost sourly. She had to reassure herself she could bring her defenses back into play. "But I still don't think that I need to gain weight."

"Why did you go back to talking about weight when we were discussing personality growth?"

"Well, I'm here to gain weight, right?"

"I'm sure that's at the top of your parents' list for your being here. Does your mother know what your father did to you?"

"I gave her hints. I would say to her, 'Don't go away and leave me with Daddy,' but she would always answer, 'Don't worry, dear. Your daddy loves you,' and leave. Yeah, he loved me all right—in all the wrong ways. No, I guess I never told her directly or explicitly what he was doing. I figured either she knew and thought it was all right, or she didn't know and wouldn't believe me, or that she might actually get mad at me and say it was my fault."

"So you could get even with her by losing weight, making her feel like a failure as a mother, a public failure at that, everyone outside the family could see how skinny you are . . ."

"They are *both* failures!" she interrupted.

Then she stopped herself, fearing that she would start to tell the story of his incestuous deeds and become vulnerable again. It was much too early for that. This was almost too much to say during her first session and feel comfortable enough to return for a second meeting.

I defused the intensity by explaining, "You have many grievances that have to be redressed. You are owed apologies. When we've known each other longer and you feel safer with 'being safe' here, in six months we may have your parents in and I'll help you get those apologies you deserve."

"You help me . . . with *my* parents?"

"I am your therapist, not theirs, you know. So, would you like to schedule our next appointment?"

She looked at her watch, then up at me, and nodded. "Yes, I would."

Donna was repeatedly sexually assaulted by her father from the age of five to twelve; by the age of seven, he was raping her. She learned early in life that she was unprotected. If one is unprotected by one's parents, then one is unprotected by the world. A mental adjustment the child may make is that "All fathers do this to their daughters and there is something wrong with me for not being able to accept his behavior."

This adjustment "helps" the child continue to think of herself as having a father, which is easier to cope with than thinking of him as a harmful, bad man living in the house.

As we have seen, this type of adjustment or defense mechanism involves the use of denial, and often amnesia, and can include self-mutilation and even multiple personality disorder, in addition to anorexia nervosa.

Incest is different from the more typical family problems such as a family depleted by illness or financially strapped, a nurturing vacuum, or parental neediness causing a reversal of dependency between child and at least one parent. But incest does cause the thwarting of the basic developmental steps—attachment, dependency, and trust—that are necessary to create security in the child.

Without the security to turn to others when in distress, the child must turn inward to soothe herself. The equation might be drawn as follows:

Balance for the child

Support received by child from others equal	=	Mental health	=	Supportive energy generated by child toward others

Lack of balance

Support received by child irregular, based on achievement only, or absent	=	Mistrust of others, fear of confrontation, low self-esteem. Abnormal people-pleasing	=	Supportive energy by child toward others exceeds support received. Child discourages support from others

Incest is the strongest "insecurity creator" to be treated in therapy. For, among other reasons, therapy involves the patient giving up some of the defenses mentioned above, which means facing the incest events, and emotionally giving up many positive feelings toward the father (or other family member). Treatment of anorexia during therapy may also invite an intensification of the other symptoms mentioned for a temporary period of time.

SHELLY AND TOMMY

Incest experiences vary in intensity and damage. Shelly was thirty years old when she came into therapy. She was five foot eleven, weighed one hundred and five pounds and dropping. When I asked her if she had experienced incest, she looked confused.

"I'm not sure if it counts as incest if I wasn't assaulted. Does it?"

"Why don't you describe the experience and its frequency."

"When I was little—say five—my thirteen-year-old brother started to hug and kiss me. Then he asked me to undress. I always wanted his approval. Sometimes he seemed like my greatest fan. He paid more attention to me than my parents did. Other times he would lose his temper and tie me up and hit me. Then I was afraid of him. When he told me to undress, he was being really nice to me. So I did. He touched and poked and penetrated me everywhere, but he was kissing me the whole time. I thought that was weird, but I wasn't scared or angry. It was nice to have him be so admiring, attentive, and affectionate. He told me not to tell our parents. I agreed. This behavior continued more frequently (two or three times a week) and I was confused by it. Something seemed strange about it, but it felt good sometimes. As an adult, I can look back and say that I was aroused by his touching me."

Shelly described her reaction to her older brother, Tommy's, sexual activity with such mildness it sounded like consensual sex. If they had been the same age, we would be in a dilemma as to whether this was "childhood sex play," something more innocent than incest and often with no psychological damage. But they were not both five years old, so even though it was not explicitly assaultive, we could not relegate these events to "consensual incest." In addition to Shelly's very young age, her relationship with her brother was abusive at other times, so her fear of this thirteen-year-old boy carried over into fearful compliance when his behavior turned sexual toward her.

When she was nine years old, she made vague complaints to her mother about her brother's behavior, saying, "I think Tommy does things with me he shouldn't," or, "Tommy does things that embarrass me."

Tommy was always regarded as strange — moody and peculiar. He had temper tantrums as well as learning disabilities at school. The family system served to focus on keeping Tommy as stable as possible in a protective fashion. His parents overlooked his minor behavioral transgressions, and even when scolded for hitting his little sister or imprisoning her in a room by holding the door, the criticism was in such a light tone that Tommy did not feel the sting of reproach. Shelly thought they barely disapproved of anything he might do to her.

"They would not protect me from Tommy. They refused to see him as dangerous to me."

Shelly's mother reacted to both of her timidly offered complaints with comments like, "I'm sure he didn't mean anything by it," or, "Maybe it was just accidental." In fact, her mother never asked Shelly to clarify her complaints. There was no interest shown in "investigating" Tommy's behavior toward Shelly. Since Tommy had warned Shelly on several occasions, smiling, "Now remember, never tell Mom or Dad about what we do," she did not want to press this lost cause lest all that would result was that Tommy would be angry with her or hurt her. She made a conscious effort to adjust to Tommy's sexual behavior with her body and allowed herself to become receptive to the arousal it sometimes created within her.

As time went on, Shelly attempted to see this behavior as normal and to act as the willing participant to her older brother. He was grateful to her for her willingness and bought her presents when she got high grades in school. He constructed a chart and pasted gold stars on it to keep a record of her achievements.

On the other hand, when he was in an angry mood, he would hit her and tie her up. This happened frequently enough for her to come home from school tense and fearful of the mood he would be in. Would he be in a happy mood, meaning he would be nice to her and they would engage in sex play? Or would he be in a gloomy mood, which meant that he would threaten her, lock her in a room, or otherwise frighten or hurt her.

Gradually, Shelly began to believe that it was her responsibility to "control" Tommy's moods. By the age of seven, she remembers trying to think of what kind of things she could say to Tommy to make sure he would be in a good mood and nice to her. The safest strategy she developed was asking him, "Do you want to play?" — which, of course, referred to sex play.

Shelly grew up from five to thirteen conditioned to deal with a male more powerful than herself by placating him, and trying to please him with cheerfulness and sex play. She lost sight of her own emotional needs, subordinating them to protect herself from his angry and withdrawn moods. For a girl her age, it all happened so unconsciously and automatically that her survival behavior became her "natural" adaptation to coping with her brother. She was not in touch with any conflicts developing within.

Her parents both worked during the day and were oblivious to the activities that were going on between their children. Their main concern was their son's problems and the resulting acting out in school. Shelly was an "A" student and posed no behavioral problems either in school or at home. They occasionally complimented her on "not being a problem."

When Shelly was thirteen, Tommy asked her to have intercourse with him. While over the years she had grown accustomed to his fondling and digital penetrations, this demand represented a drastic change. They had come to view their sexual behavior as collaborative. (Shelly had adapted to enjoy the times she was aroused, which made her feel like a guilt-ridden co-conspirator.) But intercourse was out of the question for her and at thirteen years of age she protested angrily at Tommy's request. This was the first time that Tommy had been yelled at and turned down by his younger sister, who told him, "Go find somebody else for that." He withdrew from any sexual requests after that, and withdrew by degrees from Shelly herself. She was upset at this withdrawal and even tried to entice him back to his old sexual behavior. Shelly had developed few friendships during the nearly eight years of sexual involvement with her brother. It had made her feel separate from other girls, even though she was outgoing and charming and they would have accepted her as a friend.

During her teen years, Shelly became friends with girls in high school and increasingly avoided Tommy. The further apart they grew, the more clearly Shelly saw the discrepancy in concern her parents expressed about her brother as opposed to her. He was a constant source of behavioral trouble in school, though intelligence testing indicated that he was in the superior range. The discussions about Tommy that Shelly overheard ranged from pride in his intelligence to worry about his making a satisfactory adjustment to adult life, given his peculiarities. Shelly rarely overheard discussions between her parents involving her. She posed no problems.

At the age of sixteen, Shelly began to date boys. She chose surly boys, abusive boys, toughs. Her girlfriends couldn't understand the discrepancy between her choice of girlfriends and "Those boys," as her friends referred to them.

After she went off to college, Shelly dated intelligent boys, but they were all moody and abusive to her. She assumed it was normal and that it was her responsibility to talk them out of their moodiness. It was uncomfortable for her when they were abusive (sometimes, though, it made her sexually aroused), but rather than be angry at their treatment, she felt an obligation to calm them down.

Shelly married a man ten years her senior as soon as she graduated from college at twenty-two. He was from a well-to-do family, promised to take good care of her, but his personality again had a moody, devaluating, arrogant aspect. At the beginning of their marriage, she thought the usual: "Jack is a typical, masculine personality." She knew she didn't find overly sensitive, gentle young men exciting. She referred to them as "wimps" for whom she felt no chemistry. Meanwhile, Jack's family's fortune dwindled due to some

poor investments until there was no money left and the job security he had in the family business disappeared. Jack became more irritable, and verbally cruel. He wasn't affectionate at all. He refused to
have sex with Shelly. She slowly lost all the feelings of love and
attachment she had felt at the beginning of their courtship and marriage.

She came to therapy at the age of thirty—at five foot eleven and
weighing one hundred and five pounds. Her friends had told her to
seek therapy since she was in the middle of a divorce, and clearly
suffering from anorexia nervosa. Shelly didn't challenge her friends'
observations and recommendations; she seemed resigned to the
truth. She was pleasantly dressed, well-spoken, and indicated that
she had a highly responsible and well-paying job.

I asked Shelly what she expected from therapy. Her answer surprised me.

"I think that you'll probably become bored with me, ignore me,
abuse me—maybe sexually—and finally tell me that you can't help
me."

"Then why did you come here? Is that what you are seeking?"

"No, it's not what I'm seeking, but I think that's all there is out
there for me," she said in a resigned tone.

"Somewhere there must exist a ray of hope that something better
can happen to you here. You can find, and probably have found,
those other experiences without coming to therapy."

She became sad. "I'm tired of hoping and being disappointed."

Shelly then recounted the story of her childhood relationship
with her brother, her college dating, and her marriage, along with
her current divorce-in-progress. When she was finished, she
declared, "I guess that's who I am, that's what I make happen, and
in some cockeyed way that's what I'm seeking. I have no complaint
against anybody but myself. I should know better, but I'm really
afraid that what turns me on are negative qualities in men."

"You seem to have fused masculinity with abuse."

"What I *wish* to get out of therapy is to change my taste in men and to stop them from abusing me. What I believe I'll get out of therapy with you is that you'll abuse me, get bored with me, abandon me, maybe even assault me."

"Why did you come here if you have such negative expectations, or are these negative outcomes what you seek?"

"I must be doing something that causes men to be nasty to me. I just don't know if I select nasty men, or cast a spell over nice men and invite them to hurt me."

"Are there nasty men in your background?"

She laughed.

"I don't fit in with the father-as-monster scenario. My father is shy and introverted but never mean or harmful. He's an intellectual and I think that our relationship has been based on intellectual ideas that I share with him. When I was too young to be able to do this, we didn't have much of a relationship at all. When I was little or even an adolescent, I think he was more comfortable with my mother taking charge and being involved with the children. No, the only man in my early life who could be nasty wasn't even a man at all, although he seemed quite large to me at the time. He was my thirteen-year-old brother.

"The thing that puzzles me about myself is that when I realized I was uncomfortable about the sexual episodes going on between my brother and me, I was much more angry at my mother than my brother. It's only lately that occasionally I get angry with my brother, but I've never brought it up to him. He'd go bonkers. He hasn't lost any of that temper that I knew as a child, but he doesn't get physical anymore."

"Have you spoken to your mother about these incidents in their completeness?"

She looked startled. "No, I think that it would destroy both of them."

"Then you have no faith in them to handle the issue?"

"I never thought of it as 'faith in them.' They've always been able to handle everything else that's come up."

"What if after you have been in treatment for awhile and you feel safe here, and have dispelled the idea that I'll become the reincarnation of other unkind and cruel men in your past, we have your parents join us for a session where you tell them?"

"It sounds so scary."

"As scary as your gaining some weight?"

"You think that my weight has something to do with my sexual activity with my brother, and my parents not knowing or stopping it, and men who treat me abusively?"

She paused and thought over all that she had just said.

"It's embarrassing how it's all making sense, though."

"Well, let's wait until you begin to gain weight and become more familiar with this setting and we can look at other issues."

Tears were falling down her blouse. She seemed oblivious to them. "I guess there's a lot I haven't thought about, and a lot I have never talked about before."

"I'm thinking you may be feeling safer here already."

"I think I could get used to feeling safe." She smiled.

"I suspect that the kind of safety you will develop here will be more real and lasting than the 'safety' provided by your low weight."

"I hope you're right . . . hey, at least I'm hoping."

Shelly attended therapy sessions twice a week for a year before we began the process of inviting her parents to join us so that they could learn about the hidden causes of the damage Shelly was currently experiencing. During the course of that year, Shelly gained fifteen pounds. At one hundred twenty, Shelly's large frame still looked too lean but not the disfigured appearance she had at one hundred and five. She jokingly complained to me about having heavy thighs. She had tentatively accepted her improved appearance. But as with all anorexics, in this recent state of weight gain, she was nervous that once she started gaining weight, how would she know that she could stop? Might she "graduate" to overweight?

I reminded her that when she was losing weight, she was not really making decisions about her weight but following a compulsion to lose more weight. She had gained each pound not out of a compulsive drive but out of a decision to gain that pound. That recovery from the physical part of anorexia nervosa involved change from compulsive "no-choice" behavior to decisive behavior. In this case, she (or we) would decide when she had gained enough weight and she could decide to stop gaining weight at that point, while maintaining the weight she had achieved. The key here was to reframe Shelly's definition of self-control from passive (disguised as assertive by her unconscious)-compulsive, into truly decisive postures, which include making choices about her weight. This choicemaking could then be applied to an infinite number of issues in her life. Future decisions she would make would therefore be more likely to be taken in her best interest, rather than for fearful or compulsive reasons.

Shelly liked the exchange. "So if I give up my control of my weight, I will have choices about behavior and relationships that I don't have now?"

I nodded.

Shelly looked at me suspiciously. "So first I really have to give up my control to *you*?"

"Let me answer you in the worst words possible, since you are most likely to hear them that way anyway. I want you to surrender your control over to my judgment. Since you don't trust others with matters about your personal welfare, this also becomes an exercise in trust."

"Exercise, my foot! If your judgment is wrong, then you've made me fat! If your prediction is wrong about my future 'freedom,' then you've left me fat and nowhere!"

"What's your best guess about the outcome of this 'exercise'?"

Shelly stuck out her lower lip and frowned in mock resignation. "My guess, and I better be right, is that you know what you're doing. Do you realize what it takes out of me to say that?"

"Probably the same as it takes for me to suggest it."

She studied me for a moment. "Okay, we'll do it your way."

Shelly let her weight climb to one twenty-six and we both agreed that was acceptable. She got her first menstrual period that month. It alarmed her but gave her the 'credential' to say that she had gained enough. Even her body had verified it.

"I know that it's a good thing that I got my period, but it's also sad for me because it means I officially don't have anorexia nervosa anymore, since it's one of the criteria."

We continued to work on issues that caused her to be attracted to abusive men. These were the only men who aroused her, and she was confused by her rational desire to find a stable, kind man she could view as masculine without the abuse and instant attraction she would find in a man who gave off abusive "vibes." We analyzed this fusing abusive behavior, feeling both valuable and desirable, to her relationship with her brother. His "rules" went unchallenged at home, so she incorporated them as truth. She then went on and transferred them to boys and men she met long after the sexual involvement with her brother stopped, as did their closeness. We had mentioned this "fusing" as an interpretation earlier, but that was merely our blueprint for "working it through," which means it changes from an intellectual idea to a real feeling and belief.

As our first year of therapy was coming to an end, we discussed bringing her parents into an additional meeting. They would have to be told Shelly's history and the resultant feelings she experienced toward them, and the damage it had caused, as well as experiencing their reactions to such information. This would be our initial step in healing the family from its very limited communications with each other.

Her mother entered the room first and stopped, puzzled by choice of chairs or couch. She looked at me for advice as to where to sit. I indicated, "I sit in the swivel chair, everyone else can sit where they choose."

Both parents chose to sit side-by-side on the couch, with Shelly on the overstuffed chair perpendicular to the couch. They were both Canadian, born in Toronto with roots in highly placed families in British society. Shelly's father was a bit of a rebel; after some business problems in Toronto, he had come to the United States and applied for American citizenship. They were both attractive, with a proud bearing, despite the tension they expected in an American therapist's office. One might have mistaken them for English aristocrats right off the plane from London. He was in his early sixties, with gray wavy hair, firm jutting jaw, tweed jacket patched at the elbows. She was about five years younger, dressed in a long, conservative silk dress, belted. She wore an Hermés scarf that reflected better economic times for both of them.

Shelly began her story, explaining, "I know that I've talked about my therapy with both of you to some degree. I've asked you 'into' it because there are some things I could not say outside this office. When I was younger—much younger—things happened between Tommy and me, sexual things."

They looked steadily at their daughter, jaws clenched, determined not to interrupt her or behave defensively until she had finished and invited them to speak or question her. Their looks were intensely focused on what she was saying but not flinching. It was admirable.

Shelly was visibly tense, yet determined to continue. There would be no stopping until everything was said.

"It began on our vacation, when I was five and Tommy was thirteen. We shared a bedroom. Tommy thought that it would be neat if he could 'explore' me. He made it sound like an adventure and he would admire me for joining him in this adventure. I was embarrassed when he took my pajamas and underwear off, but he kept kissing me, and being nicer than I ever remembered his being to me. I guess I decided it was worth the embarrassment to get such nice behavior from him. After the vacation was over, he waited for me to come home from school and at least three times a week 'explored' me. At first it was all on the outside of my body, then it was on the inside." Shelly stopped for a minute, looked down at the carpet, tears streaming onto her blouse and skirt though she didn't acknowledge them. She took a deep breath and resumed.

"I knew that I couldn't talk about this to my friends. I never really got close to the other girls at school or in the neighborhood because, well, I believed I had a secret which would be unacceptable to tell them and Tommy was taking up so much of my time with his 'exploring,' which left me less social time. I was afraid to invite other girls to the house. I didn't know whether he would explore me in front of them or try to explore them. The hardest and worst thing about it at the time was that . . ." Shelly broke down, sobbing. It stopped her talking for two minutes.

Her parents kept their silence, paralyzed by this new information. Shelly began speaking again though she was still sobbing. "The worst thing about it at the time was that I enjoyed it sometimes. His admiration, niceness—and even physically." She collapsed. Her mother got up from the couch. Leaning over the side of Shelly's chair, she hugged her daughter and patted her on the back, the way one would a child who was frightened.

Her father's eyes widened. He put his hands up in the air in rage and frustration and in a loud voice, which became more British as he continued, spoke for the first time.

"It's all our fault—we were asleep at the switch. We should have never let them share a room on a vacation! We neglected Shelly's safety!"

Suddenly, he began to cry. He put his head down into his hands. Now all three were crying. I came pretty close myself. The sadness was palpable, as if the walls were crying along with this family.

"But, darling," Shelly's mother implored, "you never told us. We would never have allowed this to go on!" Her mother shook her head from side to side as she spoke as if to chase all this horrible information away.

"I didn't think that anyone wanted to know. You were always so worried about Tommy because things were wrong with him—"

"Things are *still* wrong with him!" her father shouted.

Shelly mobilized some of her anger. "Well, *he* was the focus. He had to be looked after! I said things to you, Mother, but you couldn't hear them. You couldn't afford to. One child was so much trouble, maybe you were afraid to hear what I was saying because you were afraid to make him worse. Maybe two troubled children would be too much for you. I thought about this when I was eight. I told you that things were going on between Tommy and me that shouldn't be. You shrugged it off. You didn't want to know. You were Tommy's protector. I don't blame you. I did then, but even then only half-heartedly—it was easier to blame myself for having difficulty adjusting to Tommy."

Just then her father interrupted. "Why isn't Tommy here now? Shouldn't *he* be part of this discussion?"

"I could never have said any of this if he were here now." Shelly began to cry again. "I could barely tell you."

"Well, we'll take care of this," Shelly's father said as if he were about to confront his son imminently.

I interrupted. "Perhaps this family repair should continue where it belongs, here."

"What do we tell Tommy about what happened here?" her mother inquired. "He knows that we're having this meeting. He even said the strangest thing to me. When I told him we were going to have this meeting, he asked me if I still loved him. He knows something is up."

I answered, "Tell Tommy if he wants to know what happens in family therapy, he must attend our meetings."

"What if he refuses?" Shelly's mother shot back.

"Then he should not be told about what happened here and we will deal with these problems without him."

In subsequent weeks, Shelly reported that her mother answered her brother's inquiries about the session as I had suggested. This apparently was the first occasion on which he had to deal with his mother when she refused to grant his wish or explain herself to him. He repeated the question he had asked before the first session (which apparently he had dreaded): "Mom, do you still love me?" She retorted, "Why do you ask that question?" He frowned and said, "Never mind."

Shelly's relationship with her mother had changed drastically, for the better. Her mother called her every day, asked how she was, and requested another session with me so that Shelly could talk about how Tommy's sexual behavior had affected her afterward. Shelly agreed and asked for a second session with her parents. This time, Tommy was invited. He refused and explained that he wanted to see me alone before he would meet with the entire family. I responded (via Shelly's mother) that I could not meet with him alone since I was Shelly's therapist, but he was welcome to join us. He refused, but persisted in asking what went on in the first session. Shelly's parents continually refused to answer.

When the second session began, everyone was less tense. Mystery and threat were replaced by a sense that we were all meeting to solve problems without any desire to harm anyone.

Shelly talked about how she sought out abusive men (her father covered his face). She tried to explain to her parents how this had resulted in a mistaken and failed marriage. She talked about how she was vigilant about avoiding her past patterns and trying not to confuse abuse with masculinity. She admitted that it was a struggle to change her attraction to men she was accustomed to, but she would be with no man until she worked this out. They cheered her on and discussed that they had changed their pattern of calling their son every day and become more constructive and supportive in daily contacts for Shelly.

Shelly for her part admitted that she was enjoying her new relationship with her parents, though she did regret that they appeared to be excluding her brother. Her parents defended the shift, indicating that they were enjoying their late-life parenting spending more time with the "easier, lovelier child," and didn't feel guilty about it since Tommy could reenter a more involved role with the family if he attended family therapy sessions. They felt like they were finally behaving appropriately with him and were healthier for having made the change.

Shelly's anger toward her mother diminished until it was gone. At the same time she was changing her relationships within her family, she was seeking out different kinds of men, warmer and nonabusive.

As of this writing, Shelly has maintained a close relationship with her parents, particularly her mother. She is receiving, after the age of thirty, the kind of thoughtfulness, attention, and affection she longed for as a child and adolescent.

This has had profound effects on her:

—She feels that she has a right to her anger, when it occurs.
—She has shifted blame, hurt, and anger from her mother and her-self to her brother.
—As time goes on and her new relationship with her parents feels more natural, secure, and permanent, she will experience less anger toward her brother.
—She has the reassurance that the sexual relationship with her brother that began when she was five and he was thirteen was none of her responsibility, nor her blame.
—Her parents made a sincere apology for "permitting" what happened by not stopping it.

These profound effects on Shelly were the direct results of the necessary "corrections" of her childhood perceptions to begin to undo the damage that incest inflicts. Ideally, this "incest model" of changes and statements should have come from the perpetrator, her brother. But he never joined the family therapy discussions.

Shelly no longer needed her eating disorder to fill the deficit between the support that she gave to others and the lack of support she was receiving. It was an unusually mild struggle for her to give up the remnants of her anorexia from that point on.

She was also able to recognize the psychologically vital deficits she suffered from—lack of attachment, trust, dependency, and faith—so that even at this late stage, there would be a continuity of these new, positive elements in her relationship with her parents.

Shelly continues to work through her self-esteem, to revise her criteria for emotional and sexual attraction to men, and to preserve the progress she has attained.

EPILOGUE

I N the previous pages, we have seen different causes, or clusters of causes, that can predispose an individual toward the develop ment of anorexia nervosa. They include: societal, genetic, familial, and chemical factors, trauma, child molestation, and incest.

Usually, several factors are present when the predisposition becomes the illness. Once it is diagnosed, the reactions of those around and responsible for the sick person will determine the course of the disorder. Other factors are more difficult to control, in some cases even impossible: the age of onset at the time of illness, the length of time the illness has persisted, the resourcefulness of people in the patient's life to help her, the willingness of an adult to enter treatment, the quality of life awaiting the patient should she recover, and the presence of other psychiatric disorders at the same time.

If a patient develops anorexia at age sixty, treatment will be difficult; even at age thirty, when she may be independent and impossible to supervise, manage, or influence, it can be very hard. If the emotional and situational issues that cause the "adjustment" of the individual to anorexia aren't removed, recovery is unlikely. If she has been sick for many years, the disorder is part of her personality and it is harder to break the mold once the die is cast. When another family member is debilitated or psychiatrically sick, family life is chaotic, a divorce is in process, or a host of other destabilizing factors are at work, no single approach to treatment will help. If the individual has multiple diagnoses, all of them will have to be identified and treated. And if some are untreatable, this will sabotage the success of treatment. Schizophrenia and substance abuse come to mind in this instance.

Institutional treatment can be more useful when outside resources are not powerful enough. But it should be seen as a way to turn around the disorder, effective only if followed up by a discharge plan that provides positive emotional incentives and a supportive, yet structured environment.

Recovery statistics for anorexia remain at less than half. Parents, friends, and other helpers must understand what they are doing in fostering the characteristics of trust, dependency, and ability to receive from others. But most of the responsibility for recovery will still fall to professionals, who hopefully are interested in their patient's development, caring about their patient, and skillful in implementing that interest and caring.

Treating and overcoming this tough disorder is a tall order. Good luck!

APPENDIX A:

THE ROLE OF MEDICATION

The very word "medication" often causes conflict on the part of a patient, especially if she is an adolescent. Parents often become alarmed as well when they think of a young person needing psychiatric medication. It is wounding to both and can make them feel as if a profound defect exists in their daughter. Anorexics may fear medication because they are afraid that it will make them gain weight. They may also be afraid that their personality will be so changed by medication that they will no longer be themselves. The issues of addiction, and side effects, legitimately arise as well. Here I would like to provide a context for understanding when and why we should consider medication as a valid part of the treatment of anorexia nervosa. Nonmedical therapists should consult with psychopharmacists to determine what medications—if any—should be used.

Anorexia nervosa typically includes several clusters of emotional problems. The most common personality problems are anxiety and obsessiveness. This means that the person is more nervous than average, worries a lot, overthinks about everything she does, is very rigid about the way (and time) things are done, does not like change, and may even have repeated behaviors that have no real consequences. Examples of this include washing one's hands fifty times a day, triple-checking door locks, buttons, zippers, and meaningless touching of the corners of objects, among many others.

Many people who suffer from anorexia also suffer from depression. Depression involves the inability to feel joy, to care about one's present life or future, and even suicidal impulses. Another disorder that sometimes accompanies anorexia nervosa is self-mutilation — harming oneself by cutting or burning the skin. Further disorders may include enormous mood changes (bi-polar disorder) from friendly and outgoing to withdrawn, or from grandiosely optimistic to morbidly pessimistic.

Some anorexics present a collection of all these problems, along with feelings of emptiness, worthlessness, changeability from liking people to hating them. When these features are all present, we often diagnose the patient as having a borderline personality disorder. People with anorexia who present with such disorders need special medications to diminish their problems. This in turn helps make psychotherapy more effective in treating anorexia nervosa.

When an individual first comes to therapy with no previous psychiatric history, most of us want to get to know that person well to explore the possibility of treatment without using any medication at all. If we sense that the person requires medication in addition to therapy, our goal is to keep it minimal. But "minimal" varies enormously from individual to individual.

Temporary vs. Permanent Medication

Often individuals assume that any medication they begin to use in concert with psychotherapy, they will have to use for the rest of their lives. This is frequently untrue. Once patients' lives become more satisfying and they have overcome the symptoms and behaviors that led them into therapy, they may no longer need medication, or need less. Some patients may need medication for an indefinite period of time, but that is an issue to be decided between the patient and the therapist/psychopharmacologist (the prescribing psychiatrist). We have little in the way of statistics to help us guess in advance what the decision will be.

Medications Most Commonly Used

If the anorexic patient is continually irritable and depressed, most physicians employ the use of the medication category we call "Specific Serotonin Re-uptake Inhibitors"—commonly referred to as SSRIs. These include (by brand name) at the time of writing: Prozac, Zoloft, Paxil, Effexor, Celexa; no doubt, many more will come. Another medication, not from this group but helpful for the same symptoms, is Serzone.

When anxiety and/or panic attacks are often present, specific medications to block these painful and destabilizing feelings may be employed. They include, most commonly, Klonopin, Xanax, Ativan, Valium, and others. Those mentioned are part of a category of medications known as benzodiazepines. Unlike the first group, the body builds a tolerance for them, so such drugs must be tapered off slowly. If abruptly discontinued, the individual will experience withdrawal symptoms, including heightened anxiety, panic attacks, and other symptoms best explained to each patient by her (or his) physician. Another anti-anxiety medication that is generally characterized by minimal or no withdrawal features is Buspar.

When obsessiveness is a prominent feature, Luvox (an SSRI) or Anafranil (a tricyclic) may be recommended by the treating physician. In severely agitated patients, or those diagnosed as having "thought disorders" (a person who has difficulty organizing their own thoughts or mental processes and as a result may become severely agitated out of frustration or behave in ways that don't make sense to us), a more potent group of medications referred to as "major tranquilizers" or "neuroleptics" may be recommended. These are prescribed with caution. Their larger number of side effects must be balanced against their benefits. (This, of course, is true for all medications prescribed.) Sometimes these medications, along with others, may be combined to combat several personality features that prevent someone from improving or recovering.

The outline given above is not definitive or conclusive. It's just an introductory "peek" at some of what's available, and the most common purposes for which they are prescribed.

Everyone entering treatment always has a choice about whether or not to take a particular medication or any medication at all. The decision is something that must be negotiated between patient, therapist, and/or treating physician. Medication by itself is very rarely the solution to anorexia nervosa, but it can be helpful to some in concert with effective psychotherapy.

Psychological Side Effects of Taking Medication

Some individuals can develop what I call "passive identity," where they see themselves as dominated by their medications. This must be dealt with in therapy or they will not be able to raise their self-esteem. It becomes apparent when someone states, "My moods and feelings are merely a function of the medicines I'm taking." It is the therapist's task continually to reinforce the concept that the medication enables the patient to become her healthiest personality. That personality is not an artificial creation of the medication. *It is her own personality, when she is not impeded by mood or anxiety disorders.*

Two good general principles to keep in mind when using medication are "Only when necessary" and "Less is better."

APPENDIX B:

RESOURCES FOR ANOREXIA NERVOSA

The following organizations are available for assistance in the form of referrals, general information, support groups (depending on the organization), and other needs. These organizations have long histories of reliability. Some have changed addresses, but, as of this writing, these are their current locations.

American Anorexia / Bulimia Association (AA/BA)
    165 West 46th Street, Suite 1108
    New York, NY 10036
    (212) 575-6200 NY Office
    (800) 522-2230 Information Line
    Web site: www.aabainc.org

Anorexia Nervosa and Related Eating Disorders (ANRED)
    P.O. Box 5102
    Eugene, OR 97404
    (503) 344-1144
    Web site: www.anred.com

Eating Disorders Awareness and Prevention Inc. (EDAP)
603 Stewart Street, Suite 803
Seattle, WA 98101
(206) 382-3587 (administrative offices)
(800) 931-2237 (public information line)
web site: www.members.aol.com/edapinc

National Association of Anorexia Nervosa and Associated Disorders
(ANAD)
P.O. Box 7
Highland Park, IL 60035
(847) 831-3438
Web site: www.members.aol.com/anad20

National Eating Disorders Organization (NEDO)
6655 Yale Avenue
Tulsa, OK 74136-3329
(918) 481-4044

RECOMMENDED READING

Bell, R. M. *Holy Anorexia.* Chicago: University of Chicago Press, 1989.

Bruch, H. *Conversations with Anorexics.* Northvale, N.J.: Jason Aronson, 1995.

———. *The Golden Cage: The Enigma of Anorexia Nervosa.* Cambridge, Mass.: Harvard University Press, 1978.

Erikson, E. H. *Childhood and Society.* New York: W. W. Norton, 1950.

Garner, D. M., and P. Garfinkel, eds. *Handbook of Treatment for Eating Disorders.* 2d ed. New York: Guilford Press, 1997.

Johnson, C. L., ed. *Psychodynamic Treatment of Anorexia Nervosa and Bulimia.* New York: Guilford Press, 1990.

Levenkron, S. *The Best Little Girl in the World.* New York: Warner Books, 1982.

———. *Treating and Overcoming Anorexia Nervosa,* 2d ed. New York: Warner Books, 1997.

Minuchin, S., B. L. Rosman, and L. Baker. *Psychosomatic Families: Anorexia Nervosa in Context.* Cambridge, Mass.: Harvard University Press, 1978.

Sacker, I. M., and M. A. Zimmer. *Dying to Be Thin. Understanding and Defeating Anorexia Nervosa and Bulima.* New York: Warner Books, 1987.

Sours, J. A. *Starving to Death in a Sea of Objects: The Anorexia Nervosa Syndrome.* New York: Jason Aronson, 1980.

INDEX